LCC
1st ed.
inscribed

Jan 2006

To mike
it's not just a
book — it's
a revolution.
Anne Bissell
thank you for
helping survivors

Memoirs of a Sex Industry Survivor

Anne Bissell

Cleopatra International Publications

PUBLISHED BY CLEOPATRA INTERNATIONAL PUBLICATIONS

All of the characters and events in this book are fictitious, and any resemblance to actual persons, living or dead, is purely coincidental. No part of this book may be used or reproduced in any manner whatsoever except in the case of brief quotations embodied in critical articles or reviews. For more information, contact the publisher.

www.cleopatra-intl-publications.com

Library of Congress Cataloging-in-Publication Data
Bissell, Anne
    Memoirs of a Sex Industry Survivor
ISBN 0-9746060-0-6
First Edition
1. Juliet West – A fictional character.   2. Sexual Abuse – Fiction.
3. Sex Industry – Fiction.   4. Recovery – Fiction.   5. Mystery – Fiction.
6. Addiction – Fiction

Copyright © 2004 by Anne Bissell
FusionFiction™ is a trademark of Cleopatra International Publications
All Rights Reserved
Printed in the United States of America

This book is dedicated to sex industry survivors around the world. My name is Cleopatra Cameron, and I am a sex industry survivor. I am also a publisher. As a publisher, my goal is to provide a forum for the re-emergence of the voice of the new feminine archetype. *Memoirs of a Sex Industry Survivor* is the first book in a trilogy, and it launches the Juliet West series. Juliet West battles the silent conspiracy of shame that immobilizes women around the United States, and worldwide.

The Juliet West series is a brand new kind of mystery. The mystery of the lost female soul. This series launches a new genre for the 21st century called FusionFiction™.

FusionFiction™ is a blend of fiction and nonfiction. Some might even call it "Reality Fiction."

Prologue

I wrote this poem when I was not quite eighteen. It was 1977 and the dawning of the so-called sexual revolution.

I am the frozen rose
Transfixed inside of my own injustices, caught up in the petals of my own obsessions
I am the frigid woman girl, the cock teaser
I am a whore
I am loved for my frozen rose beauty
I am the blind bride waiting to see
I am an end to all men's worries
They look at me and forget everything but my illusion
I am a softly wailing polisher keeping within the walls
the silver bars of society.

I am the frigid prostitute
I must bloom; the ice forms from the tears of pain I cry
To live, I freeze the pain
To die would be to melt
To feel the heat, the pain
The truth.

I am your New Years Dream; that bitch who moans
on cue
Making you believe her pain is your pleasure
I give you the strength to believe in all of your resolutions
I hold my red lipped china doll face up and
Swallow a year of your contempt
I am the frozen rose and I must very weakly, very strongly
Be a broken doll vessel
Waiting for Grace.

Spring, 1999
California, USA

The online madam's message flashed across my computer screen: "My escorts make $80.00 for one hour, $120.00 for two hours, $250.00 for all night, and $500.00 for 24 hours. Would you like to escort movie stars and clients in HOLLYWOOD and BEVERLY HILLS?"

My heart pounded as I read the words again. *"Would you like to escort movie stars and clients in HOLLYWOOD and BEVERLY HILLS?"*

The word "escort" sounded so glamorous, especially when associated with cities like Hollywood and Beverly Hills. "Yes!" I typed.

"What is your current marital status?" the madam asked.

"Single," I responded, although it wasn't true. This was an example of the power of the internet. I could create an entire persona; become anyone I wanted to be. I waited for her response, feeling a surge of excitement that was strangely intoxicating.

"Please let me know your measurements, and I'll need a picture that I can download."

I told her that I was 34 years old, although I was really 40. After all, at the age of 40, one is considered ancient in cybertime, and a senior citizen in the sex trade. I told her that my bra size was 36B, even though I actually wore a 34B. And, of course, I mentioned that I was ten pounds lighter than my true weight.

"SENT," I typed on my keyboard. The picture I sent her was not taken very recently. In fact, in it, I was 20 years old, (give or take a few years). As I waited anxiously for her response, I wondered what in God's name I was thinking. And yet I couldn't stop myself.

Finally, after what seemed like an eternity, she responded. "You look like you might meet our qualifications."

I smiled as I typed. "Where is your office?"

"My office is in San Diego but I have clients all over the country."

I told myself that I was going along with our conversation only because I was a repressed novelist/poet stuck working in the computer industry. I had been trapped in the computer industry ever since I'd gotten out of college in the early eighties. As I scratched my way to the top, I continued to bump my head on the glass ceiling that kept women from truly advancing. After all, women had only been in the workforce for the last twenty years, since the dawning of the second wave of the women's movement in the late seventies. Equal rights were a long way off.

Besides, how was I supposed to come up with any new, exciting material writing hardware and software documents that no one ever even read? My conversation with the cyber madam was simply grist for the mill, a clever method for me to gather research pertaining to the sex industry. In addition, another motivating factor propelled me to continue my online discussion. Fear. I had only recently gotten married (for the third time) and things weren't going that well. I found the possibility of going through yet another divorce quite unbearable. Apparently, I had no idea how a real relationship was supposed to work. By real relationship, I am referring to a relationship in which both parties are present, in the same room, at least some of the time. In general, I have always found ways to create distance. True intimacy represents a loss of control that I find extremely uncomfortable.

Why not revert to old ways? I debated. *At least I'll be in control.* "Okay," I typed. "What's the next step?"

"Would you make a good escort? If so, why?"

I pondered for a moment, and then typed my response. "I am smart and sexy."

"Can you escort in HOLLYWOOD and BEVERLY HILLS?"

The words on the screen blurred, and I sat back in my chair.

Lost in cyber-reality, I transformed into Julia Roberts, the hooker with the heart of gold who starred in the 1990 movie *Pretty Woman*. In my fantasy, a smooth talking john who looked like Richard Gere rescued me from a life on the streets and transformed me into a wealthy, pampered princess overnight. But then my cyber dream ended abruptly. I closed my eyes and a new series of images assaulted me.

* * *

Surreal silhouettes moved towards me, groping. I was being initiated into the world of prostitution, or paid rape. Men. Different men—strangers—each one of them taking turns. I was a child. Seventeen.

One, after another, and then another.

When would it end?

I tried to tell them to stop, but they just laughed at me. It wasn't supposed to go down this way, but it did, and there was nothing I could do about it.

"*Stupid bitch,*" one of them said. "*What the hell did you expect?*"

He was right, of course. It was my fault. I deserved what I was getting. And so I just lay there. Numb. Powerless. I had no right to feel indignant—after all, I had willingly rented out my vagina to them.

It isn't really that bad, I told myself, and then the room began to spin, and everything faded to black.

* * *

Although my initiation into the sex industry had happened well over a decade earlier, when the flashback hit, it was more real than my current reality. I became the star of a horror movie that played over and over in an endless loop.

After that incident, and many others like it, I never really was the same person. I became two girls. I began to disassociate, to split off from my true, authentic self. A tough persona took over. This "badgirl" vowed to never let anyone get to her again. She would never let me lose control again.

For many years, this aspect of my personality kept me alive. The pure innocent child of god, my true authentic self, went underground. She waited. When it was finally safe for her to come out, I reassured her that she was still innocent, untouched, and not to blame for the sexual crimes committed against her.

I will never be free of the images that haunt me, and although I am on a journey towards wholeness, I believe that some of my emotional scars will never heal completely. My only hope for complete recovery is to keep telling my story. My name is Juliet, and I am a sex industry survivor. I am one of the lucky ones who made it out alive. I became as addicted to the power and control I mistakenly thought I held over my johns, or tricks, as an alcoholic is to their first drink.

I turned my first trick when I was seventeen. It was 1977. I got out of the sex industry in 1981, when I was 21. I carried my secret for over a decade. Then, in 1991, I met a woman who admitted to being a prostitute. Since then, I have been sharing my story with other sex industry survivors. Since then, I have been trying to understand the interrelationship between sexual abuse, incest, and prostitution. This is my mission…my quest…I am here to expose the connections between these sex crimes. I am here to tell the truth, so that other survivors might find strength in my example, and will become empowered to break out of patterns of victimization.

"WHERE DID YOU GO?" prompted the indignant online madam, in bold red type. "DO YOU WANT TO BE MY NEXT STAR?"

"Maybe not this time," I typed on my keyboard, and then signed off of my online mail service.

I wondered, as I shut my computer down, how I could have entertained, even for a moment, the idea that somehow it might be okay for me to dabble in sex work again. For a moment, I had forgotten the depths of depravity, humiliation and despair I had experienced as a prostituted woman. I had conveniently displaced the truth. The truth? That by entering the sex industry I had taken a shortcut that nearly cost me my sanity, my soul, and my very life.

For a moment, I had been lured in by three simple words. *ESCORT. HOLLYWOOD. BEVERLY HILLS.* The online madam no doubt recruited women all over the country with those three words alone. I thought of my friend who had a fifteen-year old daughter with access to the internet.

The girl's father, a drug addict and sexual abuser, had abandoned her when she was only six. And now the teen was beginning to act out. She had developed a reputation in the small Texas town that mother and daughter lived in. She was loose, easy—a slut.

One day, perhaps she might read the online madam's invitation to enter the sex industry. With just a touch of the keyboard on the madam's computer, bus tickets could be magically produced, and with the blink of an eye, the confused teen might board a Greyhound Bus en route to "Beverly Hills," or "Hollywood."

When the teen got off the bus, there would be many job opportunities open to her, and not just turning tricks. In fact, the actual act of sex for money, or common prostitution, comprises only a small part of the multi-billion dollar, worldwide, multi-racial, commercial sex industry.

The commercial sex industry includes prostitution, madaming, pimping, pornography (modeling, production, distribution, sales outlets, movie houses). Activities that commercialize the sexual fantasy are also part of the sex industry. These include stripping, phone sex work, bondage and discipline clubs, live sex shows, and internet sex sites.

With any luck, my friend's daughter would make it out of the sex industry alive.

For nearly twenty years I have studied women in the sex industry. Their stories became a mirror, reflecting back my own fractured, split self. Together we wandered through the forbidden maze called the sex industry.

The prostitute is an archetype. She is the perfect metaphor for feminine evil. She has become a scapegoat for our sexual shame, that ancient puritanical cloak we still wear. We blame her for this unresolved shame. And since she is to blame for possessing sexual qualities we cannot control, we cast her into non-human status.

Everyone knows that you are either a good girl or a bad girl, a whore, or a Madonna. This dualistic paradigm of female sexuality has created a split, a schism in our collective consciousness.

Good girls deserve to live, bad girls must die. This fact is best illustrated by the mortality rate of women in the sex industry. If a woman is not murdered, she may pick up deadly diseases. And yet we tend to discount these casualties to the sex trade, believing that these women asked for it. They were prostitutes. *What did they expect?* We place them in a role. They were bad girls—bad girls who might be your sister, your daughter, your mother, your girlfriend.

There is a double standard for men and women involved in the sex industry. For example, while male porn performers are heroes, female porn actresses are chewed up and spit out like clockwork. And even if they do become "stars," they can never go home again.

And there is a psychological aftermath to life in the sex industry that is similar to post-traumatic stress disorder. To survive in the sex industry, a part of me split off. I will never be at home in my own body, not completely. The sex industry is ravaging to a woman's soul.

I was both voyeur and participant as I pursued my scientific study of women in the sex industry. While I attempted to heal my own split consciousness I conducted research. *I do not recommend this procedure to anyone.* Once you are in the sex industry it changes you. You bite into the myth of feminine evil. The consumption of the rotten apple of sexual shame can kill you.

That night, hours after my discussion with the cyber-madam, I had a nightmare. In this recurring dream, a man is hunting me down and trying to capture me. After he molests me, he gives me money and tells me I better not tell anyone. I first became aware of the nightmare after I became clean and sober from drugs and alcohol in 1987. I thought the dreams had stopped when, in the early 90's, I confronted my stepfather about the sexual abuse that had taken place in my home from the time I was five until I started running away as a teenager.

But the nightmares had not stopped, and I woke up covered with sweat. Faces…faces looming over me, I am powerless, helpless. Would I ever be free of the images that haunt me?

Once again, I would have to look back to my past. I would have to hunt for clues. I knew there was an interrelationship between childhood sexual exploitation, prostitution, and my current life. I would have to keep digging for the truth. I would have to go back, back to 1991, when I first told my dark secret. I needed to figure out why, after so many years of freedom from the bondage of addiction to the sex industry, I could still be lured in by flashing messages:

WOULD YOU LIKE TO ESCORT MOVIE STARS IN HOLLYWOOD AND BEVERLY HILLS?

chapter one

There are good girls and there are bad girls the only difference between them is that bad girls can never go home . . . I am telling my story for all the scared little girls who made the wrong choices and went down the wrong path.

Ten years ago I was a prostituted woman. It was 1981, and I was 21 when I left that life behind. Now I am 31. At the time I referred to myself as a call girl, which made my involvement in the sex industry sound glamorous.

But now, as I look back, I can see that what happened back then had nothing to do with glamour. Instead, it was a betrayal of my innocence and that special bridge of time between adolescence and adulthood. Perched precariously on this bridge, I almost lost it all—my soul, my ability to trust, and my very life. Since I became a prostitute before the legal age of eighteen, I was a child prostitute. Or, more accurately, a prostituted child.

It all began with the knowledge that men had power and that if I could get them to desire my body I could control them and get some of their power. My body betrayed this knowledge, and at the old age of sixteen I was convinced something was wrong with me. I was convinced that I would never have an orgasm. Every time a man touched me I became so terrified that I called myself the frozen rose.

During the seventies it seemed everyone wanted to talk about women's new sexual freedom. Women were now free to express themselves, free to have as many lovers as they wanted to, and free, most importantly (or so it seemed to me), to have orgasms.

There was something horribly wrong with me though. I had never had an orgasm, let alone multiple orgasms. And even though I was only a teenager, my sexual performance left me feeling inadequate. Everywhere I looked there was some discovery that would change a woman's orgasmic power forever, such as the controversial publication of the Shere Hite report which announced women did not always climax through the missionary position.

Countless books and magazines on orgasms also became popular. These books described in detail the art of both giving and receiving orgasms. I grew up surrounded by these books. My stepfather, a sex addict and scholar on the topic of human sexuality, kept our bookshelves well-stocked with books on similar topics.

To compensate for my apparent orgasmic deficiency, I went on a quest. I became a nymphomaniac. A nymphomaniac is described as someone with abnormal and uncontrollable sexual desires. I was always hearing bits and pieces about myself that didn't quite fit together. That brazen, nymphomaniac, self-destructive person they described—it couldn't be me.

I am going to tell a story about what it's like to be so entrapped in the bad girl maze that you nearly lose your life. Only by telling you these experiences can I then reclaim myself. I believe that when you are the victim of early childhood exploitation, the emotional aftereffects can stay with you a lifetime.

I also believe there is no such thing as good girls or bad girls. It's more like lost girls, sad girls, hurt, broken or wounded girls. Girls who were sexually violated at an early age. Girls who find a way to repeat that original violation, and then become locked into destructive patterns that they believe they are powerless to change.

I was locked into destructive patterns even after I had been out of the sex industry for many years. I picked abusive men who reinforced my feelings of shame and unworthiness. I sought solace from raging husbands, unwittingly fleeing into the arms of lovers who turned out to be equally abusive. I became entrenched in sexually addictive patterns which were both damaging to my self-esteem and life-threatening. Why was I still acting out the same behaviors? Was I simply a loose female—a slut? I believe my personal experience in the sex industry is a reflection of the mythology still shrouding women as we enter the new millennium.

During the seventies, a sexual revolution swept through the United States. For some, it might have meant pleasure and liberation. For me, the so-called revolution catapulted me into a lifestyle I was not ready for. I felt pressured by society and by just about every man I encountered to be sexual. And I really didn't think I could say no, or that I had the right to set sexual boundaries.

And yet I felt blamed for being too sexual. I was, after all, a nymphomaniac, a slut. I believe that as a culture we sexualize girls far too early. Before she is mature enough to be able to adequately protect herself, she may be subjected to molestation, harassment, exploitation, and rape.

In my own lifetime, I went through all of that, and more. Before I was even eighteen I had been incested by a family member, molested by countless strangers, and gang-banged by a group of johns. As a prostituted child, I sold my body, sometimes exchanging sexual favors for a meal, a place to stay, or cold, hard cash.

I gave away something precious so often that I learned to deny my own shame. I told myself I didn't care what people thought of me. Besides, deep down I believed I deserved to be whispered about, shunned, and ultimately isolated and rejected.

* * *

June 1991
Southern California

Patrick and I were leaving San Diego to visit his parents on the Central Coast. Patrick and I were planning to get married.

"Look at that god-damned hooker over there," he hissed.

"What are you talking about? What the hell—Patrick, you just went through a red light."

"I can't believe you didn't see her," Patrick said.

"The only thing I saw was my life passing before my eyes—you just missed hitting that car by a split second."

"That cop ought to just take her out and shoot her."

I looked behind me. I could barely make out the outline of a cop, and a woman dressed in shorts. Since it was summer, the shorts didn't necessarily indicate that she was a prostitute. "How do you know she's a hooker?"

"She's a god-damned whore." He spat out the word "whore" with such contempt it felt like a bullet headed right for my heart. It was as if he had uttered those condemning words to me.

"It's like this," he explained, taking the onramp that lead out of downtown San Diego to 5 North. "A nice girl deserves to live, a whore does not."

And there it was. My future husband believed, with every cell of his masculine being that this girl did not have the right to exist. Maybe you're wondering how I even dare talk about my former profession. Or maybe you don't care. You might even feel secretly disgusted, like my future husband, who believes whores are contemptible.

Until recently, until I began to tell the truth about my past, I agreed with the emotions surrounding his contempt. I felt the whore/girl I had been never should have existed. I forced her underground. I pretended that all she had been through had never happened.

For ten long years I kept her a secret. I wanted to stay alive, after all. I knew what people would say about the whore child I had been. I knew what people would think. But deep in the abyss of my unconscious mind she roamed, waiting impatiently to be released, begging to be recognized. She whirled inside of me, dancing, flailing about, darting into my dreams at night, so out-of-control this whore/girl.

Finally, the heat from her dancing penetrated the subterranean levels of my consciousness. At first she chanted in the cavernous chasms of my cells, waiting, desperate to be released. But then the chants became howls.

Listen to my story, she demanded.

One way or the other, the truth just has to come out.

Before it's too late.

Listen...

Patrick and I didn't say much as we headed down the California coast to San Luis Obispo, where his parents lived. Biting my lip as I peered out the car window, I knew I would have to tell Patrick about my past. But how could I tell him something that would make him hate me—that would change how he felt about me before we even walked down the aisle?

I was beginning to get very nervous, if you want to know the truth. My stomach felt all knotted up inside, and I told myself that surely I must be carsick.

"Patrick," I said timidly.

"That's my name."

"What if, well..."

"What?"

"Well, how big of a wedding do you think we should have?" I asked.

"I don't know."

"Have you thought about the kind of music we should have at the reception?"

He never did answer, which didn't seem to be a very good omen.

I'm sitting in the back yard of my fiancé's parent's house. We drove from San Diego into San Luis Obispo late last night, having survived nightmarish Los Angeles traffic, drive-by shootings, and an onslaught of lemons, apparently overly ripe, that spilled from the back of a truck and danced helter-skelter onto the four-lane highway.

I've always found it ironic that Los Angeles is called the city of angels—LA, the city of serial killers, street gangs, rock cocaine and staggering air pollution. But here, in the sheltered haven of this suburban back yard, I shouldn't be concerned about such atrocities. I should feel peaceful and content, but I don't.

In the near distance, I hear the voices of Patrick and his father; they are involved in a heated conversation on the fine art of insurance adjusting. I met Patrick in an Alcoholics Anonymous meeting over three years ago. I hadn't had anything to drink in over a month. Patrick had not had one for a week.

I looked across the room and saw this angry looking man, scowling at the floor. I knew right then and there that he was the one for me. I have since learned that I picked men like Patrick because secretly I feel that I deserve to be punished. Also, he was damned good looking. The truth is, I'm addicted to love, just like I'm addicted to alcohol, money, and I guess prostitution.

But that's a lot to take in. We'll take this one step at a time.

As I mentioned earlier, I haven't been in the life for over ten years. Just so you know, prostitution is often referred to as "the life." Although I try not to think about the past much anymore, it still hurts. I made some bad decisions back then, most of them based on fear.

Funny what a little desperation will make you do.

A big black crow swept down and landed on the fence, his beady eyes peering suspiciously at me. I flapped my arms and the crow darted off, cawing indignantly. All of a sudden, I felt hot, and the faint summer breeze did me little good. I was beginning to feel a little claustrophobic. Maybe I needed to go to an AA meeting.

I guess I've always been restless. It hurts too much to stick around in one place. Even at ten, I moved fast. Once, on Easter Sunday, dressed in a blazing pink dress, I ran so fast that I tripped in the church aisle. When I looked up, the churchgoers glared suspiciously at me, as if I had done something horribly wrong.

It was a belief about myself I internalized.

YOU ARE A BAD GIRL!!

YOU DO NOT BELONG HERE!!

Years later, my mother told me that my stepfather had turned to her in church that day and said, prophetically, "She'll run away at sixteen."

I ran away the first time at fourteen; then again and again after that, from the East coast to the West coast, back and forth, and back again, sometimes with no more than five dollars in my pocket. Greyhound buses, trains, and 747 jets were my homes.

Sometimes I wonder if I've ever stopped running away—from life, from feelings, from an inexplicable sadness—and a longing to express all the things I've kept hidden for so long. So much of what I did in my life was to avoid the storm of pain locked inside. And so I drank. Or I shoplifted. Or I had affairs. Anything but feel the feelings.

Gazing out into the distance, I studied the sun-scorched hills, and I thought about the precarious nature of Southern California. You lived daily with the threat of earthquakes, fires, mudslides and various other natural disasters. Often it was a case of a near miss, such as the 7.2 earthquake that took place last week. Fortunately, the earthquake's epicenter was at the bottom of the ocean.

Next time you always thought, next time we might not be that lucky and all of California might vanish. I guess the truth is, what we all believe to be true can change in the blink of an eye. It was weird that I was thinking such apocalyptic thoughts. I mean I should feel safe here in this perfectly all-American suburban home.

This is where Patrick grew up. It was in this very home that Patrick received his "How To Be a Boy" lessons. Back when he was growing up, the nuns used to slap his eager wrists with rulers, and when he told his mom about it, she would ask him what he'd done to deserve it and hit him again. Needless to say, he has a little anger towards women. But I'm thinking that will all get worked out once we say our "I do's."

One more time, I was starting to feel a little apprehensive. I felt slightly sad too, and there was a dull ache right around my heart. I tried to convince myself that I was simply jittery about our upcoming wedding, but the real story was that I was terrified about telling Patrick the truth.

The truth about me being a whore. Oh, excuse me, a "call girl." It really doesn't matter what you call it, because everyone's opinion is still the same. Whores, prostitutes and even call girls are evil. You know what I think? I believe that when we label women either good or bad, whore or Madonna, virgin or prostitute, we trap them in a maze and a myth.

But I'm not really sure that Patrick would want to hear all about all that. He's Catholic, after all, from a fine upstanding Irish-Catholic family. In fact, his mother, Mary, has pictures of Jesus and the Virgin Mary all over the place. And even though Jesus was pretty understanding about the prostitution thing, I'm not so sure Patrick or his family members would be. But no matter what his reaction might be, I had to tell him. And I had to tell him soon.

Pensive for a moment, I thought about Patrick's family. They are fine people; they are sturdy, normal and purposeful. Do they really believe I'm a nice, suitable future bride for their only son? Pondering the obvious impropriety of a nice Catholic boy like him hooking up with a fallen woman like me, I then start thinking about my childhood.

My father ran off with a Japanese woman when I was nine months old, so I didn't exactly have a father figure. Technically, she wasn't a woman yet—in fact, she was our sixteen-year old baby sitter. I didn't find out about the part where she was our sixteen year old babysitter until a few months ago. Somehow it made everything I understood about my father even worse.

My father's career as a writer was interrupted by visits to various California vacation stops, otherwise known as prisons. Besides, he gave up on working when he was in his early thirties. One day, his wife, in a drunken stupor, told me that my father was an heir to a mattress company that had been owned by one of his four stepfathers. I don't know how much money was involved, and maybe that's not the point.

The point is, of course, that if he had all that money, why didn't he spend some of it on his family? It was bad enough to have a career criminal for a father. But a career criminal who apparently stole just for the thrill of it made no sense at all.

My father always lived at least 3,000 miles away, and therefore, he could not protect his family. Everyone knows that little girls need to be protected from the wolves and child molesters who roam the streets. Besides, if he had been around, maybe he would have stopped me from wearing hot pink to church that day. After all, good little girls do not wear hot pink to church. Or perhaps he might have taught me that all important Perfect Girl strategy called "The Art of Saying No."

Standing outside in the backyard, I couldn't help but overhear, through an open window, Patrick, who, along with his father, continued to be caught up in a rambunctious discussion. Upon closer inspection I saw that the entire family had gathered around the dining room table. I went back inside to see what was going on.

Whenever we visit Patrick's family, I am reminded of all the experiences I missed out on as a child, such as a family that actually did things together—you know, simple things, like playing a card game such as the one they were all involved with right now. Each of them appeared so excited as they slapped cards down. They were a family, and each of them knew without question that they belonged.

Not being much of a card player, I sat on a nearby sofa, trying to complete a crewel embroidery piece I had been working on for almost a year now. The front part of my tapestry was a lovely flower arrangement. On the other side, there was a tangled mess of multi-colored threads.

I am sure that Patrick's family would be surprised to know that as I stitched my flowers, I was really envying them for looking like such a good family on the outside, even if in reality, they were not.

As I stitched, I wished I had been blessed with more attentive parents. And finally, as I stitched, I longed for a mother and father who had been able to tell their daughter was about to go down the wrong path.

Why couldn't I have been protected? Why wasn't I raised as Patrick and his three sisters were, in the womb of the watchful Catholic Church? While I was riding on Greyhound buses and sleeping on stranger's couches, his sisters were being taught the dangers of sex before marriage, abortion, and the problematic nature of dating non-Catholics.

Somehow, I had never learned all those girl-training rituals. Like how to sit quietly, with your ankles crossed, and mind your manners, so that people are instantly aware that you are a Good and Pure Girl who knows how to say no. Surely some of those lessons might have proved helpful to me, I thought, as I put my tapestry down and went back outside.

I paced back and forth in the small yard, and then stopped in front of an apricot tree. Above me, between the limbs of the tree, a spider has built a sturdy web. Just as the apricot tree has spider webs which link it to the spider, there are invisible webs that will forever connect me to my past.

* * *

1981
Baltimore Washington Airport

Everything will be different as soon as you get to California, I thought as I climbed aboard the plane en route to San Diego. *My past will just melt away. I'll be instantly redeemable, like a bottle of coke.* I'll fly from the East Coast to the West Coast, and leave the past behind me. I never knew that I carried with me a network of invisible webs which linked me, inextricably, to all my experiences in the sex industry.

Instead, I only felt relief. Tucked away in the momentary safety of a 747 jet, I watched dirty, grimy Baltimore disappear behind me, eclipsed by pure white clouds. I was leaving the life behind—the sex industry—that had begun to control me as heroin controls the addict.

The day I climbed off that 747, I believed I had engineered an amazing transformation. In my mind, I looked lovely, innocent, and pure. I was a fresh-faced college graduate ready to begin her new life with her future husband.

On the morning we said our wedding vows, I was hung over. The preacher's face blurred before me. I knew enough not to agree to the OBEY part. I started sobbing uncontrollably. Again, just as they had done when I was ten, the people in the church stared at me.

What's wrong with her, I'm sure they were all thinking. *Doesn't she know this is the happiest day of her life?* Here I was being rescued by Prince Charming from the depths of sleaze and depravity, and all I could do was cry. Even as we marched to our honeymoon suite, complete with a revolving bed and Jacuzzi, I couldn't stop crying. Glaring out the hotel window, I muttered pitifully, "It's like a death."

"What's like a death?" my new husband Craig said, trying to remove his cufflinks.

"Marriage," I said, makeup streaming down my face.

My husband finally got the cufflinks off, but he didn't say anything.

As far as the sex act goes, I have the distinct impression that something happened, but I'm not quite sure what. I think I was more concerned about the logistical strategies required to maneuver within all that bridal regalia: garters, stockings, push up bra, and so on.

I probably did not have an orgasm, because, although I liked to think of myself as a sexual goddess, I was actually sexually numb. Frigid could not be the term. Let's call it sexually disabled. But the perfect bride transformed into the whoregirl and you would have thought it was the sexual experience of a lifetime.

After we had consummated "The Act," we went to dinner in the hotel dining room, where this stupid girl was prancing around in MY wedding dress. Consider the odds of such an occurrence. And yet while it certainly might not have been the best of omens, our marriage was doomed from the start anyway. I had so wanted to believe that I could just leave the past behind...But in running away from the past I had picked up a few destructive habits, like alcoholism, drug addiction, and an inability to separate fact from fiction.

In short, I had no conscience. Out there on the streets you learn to take and you learn to use and you learn to not think twice about it. You feel justified in doing whatever you need to do to survive. And so you learn not to care, because caring would not be cost-effective.

* * *

June 1991
San Luis Obispo, California

And now I'm engaged to be married for the second time. Secretly I am hoping that this time I really will be able to become The Perfect Wife, and therefore, the Good Little Reformed woman.

It's strange that whenever I feel that old hurt or pain coming up, I'll think about turning a trick. It's like, the world's messing with me, I'll show them, I'll use a man, take his money, MAKE HIM PAY.

I've heard that you can take the girl out of the street but you can't take the street out of the girl. I don't agree. I think there's hope. I'm not saying that I'm Susie Goodie-two-shoes today, but I do know that it's possible to change. As long as I don't pick up a drink or a drug, it's possible for me to continue changing.

Before last week, I thought I didn't have that whore/girl in me anymore. After all, I was now, at the time of my second engagement, over three years clean and sober from drugs and alcohol. Like I already said, I met my fiancé in an Alcoholics Anonymous meeting, which is almost like meeting one's future mate in a church. For the first two years of our relationship, I was good, just like Patrick's three sisters, faithful, true, committed, each a veritable Madonna. But then last week I had this fling with this guy I used to work with.

We did it three times in a sleazy hotel. It was sad how familiar that hotel seemed. Even the smell, an orange, antiseptic fragrance, was known to me. I am an unfaithful woman. I guess I just have this inability to be completely honest with myself and others.

I won't lie about one thing—I loved having sex with this guy. Maybe it's the whore in me that can compartmentalize the moment; like a man I can enjoy sex just for the sake of it. Don't get me wrong, when I quit drinking I started working on being more honest. But then the old thinking re-surfaced. *Another man would fix me*. Either I use sex as a drug, or maybe I'm just not capable of complete honesty, or a mixture of both.

It's hard to know sometimes. Honesty was one of the "How To Be a Perfect Girl" lessons that I missed. I began to acquire early training in the art of deception from my stepfather, who was a pathological liar. He came into the picture when I was about three years old. He even lied about what time of day it was.

Webs. Webs which connect the girl I was before to the woman I am today.

You might as well get used to the idea. This book is not going to be a Harlequin Romance story. My story isn't sugarcoated, or airbrushed, or Cinderella-ish, but it's real. Perhaps you might have thought it was going to be, since I talked about crewel embroidery and all, but no, this isn't going to be a sweet saga.

So, here I am, pacing the length of this back yard in what's considered California's central coast area, San Luis Obispo. If you're ever in the area, the Hearst Castle is always a fun attraction. But anyway, you don't want to hear about that. You want to hear about how I'm here, yet at the same time, I'm also back in Baltimore because I couldn't just kill that whore/girl off.

I'm here, but I'm also still sitting in the hospital waiting room, wondering why my mother has swallowed a bottle full of little blue pills. I'm wondering why she wanted to die so much. I'm here, but a part of me, held back by those invisible webs, is gone, still laying on a hotel bed with some stranger as he does his business, that awful orange antiseptic smell wafting around us.

I'm still split into different fragments of self, which I am busy trying to collect into one unified whole. I know for a fact that I split off from myself when I was a whore. Another girl turned those tricks. It's called disassociation, but I just call it the split.

When I was about sixteen, this friend of mine, who later took the street name Penelope, told me she liked having sex with guys for money. I was shocked. I mean she was from the same white middle class neighborhood I was. She had read *The Happy Hooker,* and to her, prostitution seemed an exotic challenge.

Nobody made Penelope turn her first trick. She wanted to, just like some girls want to be cheerleaders. The first copy of *The Happy Hooker* that I ever read was the one that I borrowed from Penelope. I found it fascinating. Another book I found educational was entitled *Coffee, Tea, or Me.* In the book, horny flight attendants, just like the infamous happy hooker Xaviera Hollander, made constant sex with strangers seem fun and exciting.

I was seventeen years old when I turned my first *official* trick. I say "official" because I believe I turned tricks as early as fifteen without even really knowing that is what I was doing. With terror and amphetamines coursing through my young body, I performed the ancient ritual, a scared little girl, flesh grinding against flesh, no idea who I was with, hoping only to get this dreadful ordeal over with as quickly as possible.

Self-justification set in immediately. After all, I'd been screwing guys left and right, hoping they loved me. This way, by doing it for money, it didn't matter if they loved me, because I would get paid. That's how quickly I crossed the line. One minute I'm shocked by my friend's ambition to be a prostitute, the next I'm rolling around on the floor with some Greek guy for maybe fifteen bucks (I didn't have my fee structure established yet).

After a while, a lifestyle that once would have been shocking and unacceptable to me became normal. As time went on, I became an expert at self-justification. I had to be a prostitute to make the money to pay for my college education. I was on my own. My father was locked up, and my mother was a pill popping suicidal alcoholic.

Motivated by a fear so pervasive it penetrated every cell of my being, I honestly felt like I had to turn tricks. In the end,

I made the choices I did because I didn't think I had any other alternatives.

How can anyone judge why a girl turns tricks? Do you think I would have done it if I didn't feel terrified most of the time? There were times when I had no more than five dollars in my pocket, nothing to eat, and no place to live. Like I said, most of my decisions were based on fear.

The sun has started to slowly creep behind one of San Luis Obispo's mountain peaks. Patrick and his sisters wanted to rent a video. I talked them into viewing one entitled *Working Girls*. I guess I figured, ten years have past, I can handle seeing something like this. After all, I left that girl behind. And I think I wanted to see what their reaction to the movie would be.

We were all in the living room passing a big bowl of popcorn back and forth. One big happy family consisting of Mom, Dad, Patrick, his sisters, and me.

"How could anyone do that for money?" shrieked Loretta, Patrick's youngest sister. "That's so *disgusting*."

Patrick's mother and father, as well as his two other sisters all turned to face Loretta.

Should I break into a scintillating diatribe on my premise that a bad girl can be a good girl inside, and that the cultural perception that she is bad is due to our entrapment in an ancient patriarchal myth of feminine evil?

In my mind's eye I could picture their reaction. This nice Catholic family with morals and values so well intact. If only life had been fed to me like receiving, during Eucharist, that tiny white bread wafer know as the host, so that I could simply swallow it and accept it and know the right way. But it hadn't been, and so I watched the scene in the movie as an outsider would, not a part of this town, not a part of this family, an alien creature who wasn't even at home in her own body.

"I mean look at her," Patrick's sister went on. "She doesn't even like that guy."

Slumping into my chair I jammed another handful of popcorn into my mouth. "Can you imagine such a thing?" I offered, trying to sound casual. But no one heard me. The evil celluloid creature slithering across the screen before them had their complete attention.

The Original Sin

Their voices float in and out
My mamma backed into the corner
My stepfather
Above
She's no good, I keep trying to tell you
She's a little slut. A whore. A bad girl
I told you she would run away
Nothing but trouble.

We need to lock her up
That's what the shrink said
It's for her own best interest
Bits and pieces of their words floating around me
Someone always telling me who I was
They didn't know
The real
Me.

I was always running running from
The original sin
The first time he
Touched me
Down
There.

I didn't bleed
But my eyes were filled with tears
And then I learned to be tough
A part of me split off, and floated way above my bedroom
That part of me saved my life
One day, I thought, as I soared safe and protected
In my glass cage above
I'll show him who I really am.
He thinks I'm a bad girl?
I'll be the best bad girl there is
Well, he made my mamma and my sister
Cry every night.

He won't ever get to me like that
I'm on my own now
On the run
I'll never go back home
For what? To be called a Whore?
I am what you made me
But soon enough, I'll be back
Walking in dignity will be my revenge.

chapter two

1977
Baltimore

It was the summer of 1977. I was seventeen. I was sick and tired of my stepfather hitting on me, treating me like I was his date. He was on me like white on rice. I needed a job, and he had given my name to his friend so that he could take nude pictures of me.

His "friend" took pictures for what seemed like an eternity. He paid me twelve dollars an hour, which seemed like a lot of money at the time, but considering some of the shots were completely nude, I guess it really wasn't. His hands were shaking as he snapped the pictures. When I saw how nervous he was, I felt this surge of power. It was a power that I believed came from my sexuality.

But I didn't want to think about either my stepfather, or his friend with the unstable grip. One thing was for sure, I knew I wouldn't be able to stay here much longer. He couldn't control me, so he would want me to move out. If I wouldn't be his little girlfriend, he would find a way to punish me. I should be used to it by now. I had been on the run since I was fourteen. It was only a matter of days before I might have to run again.

I didn't want to care, didn't want to feel.

I liked to think that I was living fast as I stopped at a red light and inhaled deeply on a joint. I put out the joint and then at the next light pulled out a tiny silver box containing amphetamines. Gulping the pill down with a Coke, I caught my reflection in the rear view mirror. I knew that my face would always help me get what I wanted.

I imagined that I was a *Playboy* magazine centerfold, a golden girl with air brushed, smooth skinned beauty, whose youthful sensuality opened all doors. Centerfolds made a lot of money, and with that kind of money I could leave town for good.

I went over to my friend April's house. April was an acting student, like me. I sat out on her porch looking through the classified section. I concluded I was either too young, or didn't have enough experience for most jobs.

Inhaling deeply on another joint, I closed my eyes and enjoyed the warmth of the sun on my face. I had an extremely fulfilling fantasy life. My usual fantasy went about like this. I meet someone incredibly sexy and there is instant electricity between us. I would have intense orgasms and my whole body would shake and quiver and I would call out his name just like in *True Confessions* magazine.

My main ambition was to have an orgasm like that. Or, if that wasn't possible, any kind of orgasm would do, since I had never had one. As I previously mentioned, I called myself the frozen rose because I felt numb, or frozen, in my vaginal area. It's kind of hard to have an orgasm when your vagina feels frozen.

I was so deep into my rich, multi-orgasmic fantasy life that I knocked a glass over with my foot.

The sound of breaking glass sent my friend April scurrying back out to the balcony. "You better learn to be more careful," she said, glaring at me. "Every time you're over here you break something."

I was always high on something, and when I got high I was clumsy. I had been using drugs and drinking since I was thirteen. I was pretty much a speed freak, although anything you had would do just fine.

"Sorry," I apologized. "Who was that on the phone?"

"The doorman from the theater," April replied.

"I didn't know you were performing somewhere," I commented, genuinely surprised.

"I'm dancing over at the Gayety on East Baltimore Street."

"East Baltimore Street—isn't that the block, the place where guys go to pickup hookers?"

"Yes." April's arms were drawn tightly across her chest. "One of the dancers quit today. The doorman wants to know if I can get somebody to fill in."

"Is that one of those places where you take your clothes off?"

She nodded. "It's six bucks a show, five shows a night, plus tips. Do you want to do it?"

"But I'm a feminist!" I declared. "I can't take my clothes off in front of strangers."

"You don't even know what a feminist is. Besides, you said you were looking for work. It's a way to earn a few bucks, that's all."

"I do too know what a feminist is. My sister is one. She's even going to college to learn about the women's liberation movement."

"You know what feminists want?" April asked, without giving me time to respond. "They want power. I have found a way to have complete power."

"Through dancing?" I said doubtfully.

"Yes, Juliet, through dancing. When I'm up there on stage I'm in complete control of the entire audience."

"I don't think being a sex object, dancing without your clothes on has anything to do with controlling the audience," I said, parroting some of the concepts I had heard about from my feminist sister, Marie. "Women can't have equality if they're just sex objects."

"This has nothing to do with being a sex object," April replied indignantly. "It's an art form." She stood in the doorway between the balcony and her apartment. "You don't have to decide until four. I'm going out for a while. You can stay here if you want but I'm going to see my boyfriend. I need to pick my costume up at the cleaners too—it sure gets dirty fast. They don't sweep the floor very much."

"April, the other day you told me your boyfriend said he couldn't go out with a girl like you. What did he mean by that?"

"He's Catholic and he thinks topless dancers are whores."

My mouth fell wide open. "How could anyone think that about you? You're only trying to make your way through college, aren't you?"

April had moved into the living room. "There's a few reasons I'm doing this," she said as she slumped down into a beat up old couch, lit a cigarette and then pensively studied its glowing red tip.

"Like what?" I asked, always the curious one.

"I feel like I'm beginning to define my *own* sexuality. Isn't that the same thing as being a liberated woman?"

I shrugged, beginning to feel confused. "I'm not sure, April."

"Well I think it is. Besides, there's also a sexual revolution going on, and that's much more exciting than a bunch of angry lesbians burning their bras and calling themselves women's libbers."

"They don't all burn their bras."

"Look, when I'm dancing, *I'm* calling the shots. I get to choose what I do with my body. And besides, it's *more* than just dancing to me. I feel important when I'm up there. I feel pretty—like I'm a star. It's just like when you're in a play, everyone is looking at you.

Once you experience it, you'll know what I mean."

Maybe April was right. Maybe the women's libbers were just angry lesbians. My sister sure seemed angry all the time, and she wasn't that much fun to be around when she started going on and on about how women didn't have equal rights. "Maybe I'll go with you, but I'll just watch."

"Suit yourself," she said. "I'll be back in a couple of hours and you can let me know then."

As the afternoon sun streamed though the latticework on the balcony, it made dreamy, crisscross patterns on my bikini-clad body. Half dozing, half daydreaming, I dreamt of a beautiful theater where I was the star of the show. Dressed in a flowing, silky white gown, I was the object of everyone's attention. Bright lights revealed my glistening lips, sumptuous curves and perfectly lacquered nails. I was a perfect doll. But when it got to the part where I was supposed to take my clothes off, the fantasy ended abruptly.

Should I even consider dancing? Was it worth it? The money didn't seem all that great, but so far, summer jobs were nearly impossible for me to find. And even when I found a job, I was usually too stoned or strung out on speed to keep it. And April made dancing seem so exciting, just like a theatrical performance.

All I knew is that I did not want to go home. For what? To have my stepfather hit on me? *No thanks,* I thought. *Anything would be better than that.*

As soon as April walked in the door she immediately offered me a joint. After we were both a little out of it, April proceeded to ask me about going down to the block. "Oh, I don't know April," I said. "I need a job, but, dancing, the block . . ."

"Take another hit," April said, passing me yet another joint. "This is really good stuff."

I took a long drag and sat back in my chair. The pot was

helping to take off the speedy edge I felt as a result of the white cross tablets I kept swallowing up, like candy, for their stimulant effect.

"Just come with me," April said persuasively. "You can watch me dance. My routines are getting better and better."

"But the block—everyone knows that's the worst part of town. My parents might get mad."

"Your parents might get mad? Sounds like your stepfather wouldn't. Maybe he'd want to have his friend take more pictures of you."

I considered what she had said, and I wondered for a brief second if my mother knew he had given my phone number to his nervous friend. Probably not.

As if sensing my ambivalence, April kept at me. "Just keep an open mind, after all, we're theater majors—we have to be able to try new things. Who knows, maybe we can even write a play about our experiences."

That made sense to me, so the next thing I knew I was walking through "The Block." Baltimore's red-light district—where sailors, businessmen and the boys next door stopped for a night of anonymous pleasure—was a sex supermarket. Neon advertisements flashed on and off telling of the various pussycats, playthings and playgirls to be consumed. Barkers informed the passers-by of the women who waited inside.

Any imaginable fantasy that could be produced in female form was there: women who spin on disks. Women locked inside of glass cages. Women who lick their lips in a sensual manner when you put a quarter in a slot. And women like hungry dolls waiting to be taken off their showroom shelves.

"Hey girly girl," shouted a barker. "Need a job? Come on in . . ." Whistles, catcalls and leering stares greeted us at every turn, and I was not enjoying the attention. My heart was beating way too fast, and my palms were sweating profusely. This was a mistake.

"April, I really don't think I should have come down here."

"Oh come on," April insisted. "It's exciting—don't you feel the beating pulse of the city? It makes me feel so alive."

"My heart is beating out of my chest if that's what you mean," I said, but I don't think she heard me.

"This is it," April said. "This is where I work, the Gayety Theater."

"I never said—"

"Hey Blacky, this is Juliet."

"Well, I reckon I'm Romeo," offered Blacky. I tried not to notice that only one of his eyes moved up and down, or that he was looking at me like a tender morsel he wanted to swallow much more than the pastrami sandwich he was working on.

April and I stood under the marquee of the new Gayety Theater as she chatted with the portly doorman. Across the street the old Gayety Theater was being torn down. Its rotting facades revealed another era when burlesque was a respected art form. According to the old photographs behind the glass cases, the burlesque performers who once danced at the old Gayety Theater had colorful, flamboyant acts that sizzled with energy and romping vitality.

Back then, I thought, *maybe it really had been "an art form," as April had called it. But things were different now.* That much I could tell from studying the slick, glossy advertisements. I examined the new billboard that was hanging by the entrance:

Meet Chanel, Miss January's Scratch and Sniff Centerfold Appearing in Hustler Magazine. Totally NUDE...Totally XXX Rated

The picture of Miss January, in comparison to the women of the bygone "burlesque era," was, even to my inexperienced eye, quite another story altogether. There wasn't anything artistic about this picture. In fact, there was something horrifying about it. Miss January was handcuffed, blindfolded, and she looked like she'd been beat up.

"Do you like my picture?" Miss January herself asked, as she came rushing up to us. "I can give you an autographed one."

"Oh that's okay, I'm not going to be here long," I said.

"I wouldn't go in there *at all* if I was you," Chanel warned. "It's a hellhole. The only reason that I'm here is because I'm a prisoner."

"What do you mean?"

"I have a group of owners," Chanel explained. "One day I woke up in this mansion. All these guys drugged me and said that I was going to be the next porn star. That's how I wound up Miss Scratch and Sniff 1977—I'm a sex slave."

"Come on," April said, grabbing my arm.

"Are you *sure* you don't want an autographed picture?" Miss Scratch and Sniff shouted after us.

April pulled me into the theater before I could respond.

Inside the theater, porno movies played to an almost empty audience. Men of a variety of ages took up the front row. I noticed movement underneath their coats, as they jerked off to the images before them. *This is pathetic,* I thought.

"What did she mean?" I whispered to April. "What did she mean she's a sex slave?"

"Forget about it," April hissed. "She's just crazy." She pulled a flimsy curtain open and we climbed some creaky stairs that led to the tiny dressing room.

I pointed to a rail-thin black woman huddled on top of a cracked, marble vanity. "Who is that?" I asked. Wearing only red bikini underwear and a skimpy matching bra, the woman's beaded, oiled and braided hair was studded with gaudy rhinestone jewels.

"Her name is Sally, and she needs to wake up—now! Come on, get going, we've got a show to do," snapped April.

Dope sick, Sally finally looked up, her ebony eyes slits. "What's she doing here?" she snarled, pointing a bony finger at me.

"She's going to dance tonight," April explained.

"I only came to watch," I contested.

Sally pulled her gaunt body up. "Well you can have this place. I know why you came here. You thought you was going to take the place of that dizzy girl who just quit here. 'Oh, I can't stand the heat,' she say. Ain't that some shit, like anyone gives a damn. What kind of place she think this is, anyway? I bet the boss wanted her to give a blow job and she wouldn't. Well they can have this place. Soon as I get enough money, I'm gonna up and quit."

I turned to April, who had emptied makeup and other articles out of her purse onto the vanity shelf. "Is that true, is that why that girl quit?"

"You heard what I said girl," Sally said. "You writin' a book or sumpin? Anyone got a cigarette? I feel sick as a dog." Sally accepted the cigarette from April. "I don't know whatchu thinkin' bringin' this girl here."

"Like I said, she's going to dance. She'll probably wind up being the star of the night," April replied enthusiastically.

"No, I'm *not* going to dance," I said. "I'm just going to watch."

"Star for the night," Sally snickered. "Yeah, an' I'm Aretha Franklin."

"Whatever," April shot back as she slid into her dance costume. First she pulled on a black g-string, black stockings, and a garter. I watched with rapt attention as she then climbed into a shimmering, clinging dress. It was just like the dress I had visualized in my fantasy.

Maybe she was right—maybe it was just like a theatrical production.

"What you starin' at girl, ain't you never seen a stripper get dressed? Getting undressed now that's the key," smirked Sally, revealing the gold cap on her front tooth.

I sat down next to Sally. "You guys should get paid more than six bucks a show."

"If you think you can do better somewhere else, then go. But believe me, it's the same ol' shit anywhere on the block. Ain't no use stayin' around this place anyway. This place ain't nothin' but a stinking rat hole," concluded Sally.

Blacky, who was now smoking an after lunch cigar, entered the dressing room. "You ladies ready? The show starts in five minutes. Hey girlie, what should I announce you as?"

"She don't think the money is good enough for her," snickered Sally.

He smiled and shrugged his shoulders. "What the hell did you expect—this ain't Vegas, and you sure ain't no pro. I'll call you Rose, okay?"

"No, that is, oh, it's just that, I don't know if I can do this!"

Blacky shrugged and walked away.

"April, are you listening? I said I don't think I can do this. And it isn't just the money. I can't take my clothes off in front of strangers."

April ignored me as she lined her blue eyes with black kohl and her lips with dark red lipstick.

"But if I don't do it, I'm afraid I'll lose our friendship."

She looked at me disdainfully and at that moment I knew I would probably go through with it, if for no other reason than to please her.

Just then, April grabbed a vial out of her purse. "Take a blast of this, and don't worry about it."

The music pulsed like a heartbeat, and I shivered with excitement as I watched from backstage. Sally danced now, and she reminded me of a snake slithering across the stage, her dark oiled skin glistening underneath the spotlight.

Donna Summer's husky voice had become one with Sally's movements: "Love to love you, love to love you baby . . ."

But even the music and the lights could not hide Sally's boredom and utter detachment from her dancing. On automatic pilot, her glazed eyes never connected with the audience as she spread her legs wide apart and began to touch her private parts.

I was shocked. There was no way I could do that. Why didn't I just turn and run? It wasn't too late. *But maybe it would be fun,* I told myself. *Like acting in a play.* No, that wasn't it—I had to leave—I had no business coming here.

Then April offered me another blast of cocaine. The mixture of amphetamines, pot and now the coke gave me false courage.

"It's your turn now, Juliet, get out there," April said.

Adrenaline coursed through my veins.

Everything beyond the foreground of the stage swarmed before my eyes. The men in the audience all blurred together into one amorphous gray mass. I went into instant disassociation; my stepfather had trained me well.

I moved quickly, terrified, hoping that if I moved quickly enough they wouldn't even see me.

"Take your clothes off," coaxed April from backstage.

"Take it off," yelled the men in the audience.

It doesn't matter, I told myself. *It'll be just like when I posed for those nude pictures my stepfather's friend took. I can just pretend I'm somebody else.*

"Take it off," yelled the men in the audience, more persistently this time, as if they were getting mad.

You aren't even really here, I thought. *Or, if I am, I'm just acting in a play.* I fumbled with the straps on my bathing suit. As the straps came down further, the men in the audience cheered even more.

I spun around like a top—faster, faster, hoping that if I danced quickly enough I might become invisible.

"Come on, quit wastin' our time," said someone from the audience. For the first time, I peered past the glaring lights and looked at their faces. I could see that they were busy...busy jerking off underneath their coats. I felt like I was going to be sick.

Horrified, I ran off the stage, and into the dressing room. There were tears streaming down my face. I grabbed a bottle of Peppermint Schnapps someone had left on the counter and swallowed. I felt the burn in my gut, felt my shame subside.

I peaked out to the stage where April was dancing now. What I saw next horrified me even more. There was my friend, touching herself on stage, moving her hands in and out of her bikini underwear, driving the men wild. She seemed to be enjoying herself, although I just couldn't understand that.

There was something very, very wrong about all of this. I had to turn away; I couldn't stand to watch her humiliate herself. But then she didn't think it was humiliating, she thought it was art or something.

When she finished her routine, the X-rated movies were instantly switched back on. There would be no other dancers tonight, only the endless images of women spinning on disks, locked inside of glass cages, licking their lips, women like hungry dolls waiting to be taken off their shelves. Objects.

We all dressed silently. For a moment, I stared with open curiosity at the small X tattooed on Sally's upper thigh. I sat down next to her. "You guys made that look so easy, but I was terrified."

Sally snorted. "You looked like you was," she said, chuckling as she pushed a loose comb into her black hair.

"You moved so fast I thought you were going to spin right off the stage," said April.

"I guess I don't have the moves like you guys do," I said.

"Long as you got a thang don't matter how you move. That's all they come here to see. Is one of you drivin'? I need a ride. No, wait a minute, I been evicted. I gotta stay with my old man so I'll just walk," Sally grumbled.

Cardboard stick figures in the front row of the theater watched drearily as the evening's live entertainment passed through. Only moments before we had been their fantasy girls, their dream goddesses of the night, and for a few precious moments, surged with hot sexual feelings, they had felt like men. Now their eyes floated back to the screen, waiting, hoping for that next fix.

As we left the darkened theater, I had the feeling that I had just woken up from a bad dream. We stopped in the lobby where April pointed out dozens of photographs of famous burlesque dancers who once danced at the old Gayety Theater.

"They used to put on a real show," she told me. "The art of strip tease, or burlesque was considered an art form."

"So what happened to it—why don't the dancers use costumes like this anymore?"

"Pornography created a different market. Look over there," she said, gesturing towards the building across the street. "The old Gayety Theater where the burlesque dancers performed is being demolished."

Across the street, bulldozers had begun to plow through the once grand building. Around this heap of concrete and scaffoldings a neon jungle pulsed with a different kind of action. A chubby, pasty-faced barker with checkered pants and alligator skin shoes whistled at us as we walked by. A girl who looked even younger than me wearing pigtails and licking on a lollipop stood in a doorway. A cop jostled a drunk who lay sprawled on the sidewalk.

April paused to light a cigarette in front of an adult bookstore and then continued walking.

"Do you know a lot of the dancers at the Gayety?" I asked.

"A few of them. There's this one woman who dances sometimes; her name is Kitty. If you ask her what she does she won't tell you. I guess she's ashamed," April said. "You were ashamed—weren't you?"

"Yes."

"All the women are ashamed deep down. Kitty told me all women who dance are as good as whores."

"Do you believe that?"

"Kitty said you learn where the real money comes from or you don't survive. She got fired from this other place because she wouldn't go down on the boss."

"Is that why the other girl quit, the one that complained about the heat?"

"Yeah, I think so."

"But that's disgusting, April. I mean, going down on some guy, just to keep your job."

"Oh, there's a way around all that," April said dismissively. "Besides, I just *love* being on stage. When I'm up there, I'm in control, and I feel like I'm it, you know—larger than life."

"Yeah, but what if you have to go down on the boss, like that girl?"

"You ask too many questions."

Next time, I vowed to myself, next time I went on stage, I would be like April. I would be in control. I had not been in control this time, and I would never allow that to happen again.

My friend April was just a small town girl from Pennsylvania. When her act was over at the Gayety, the movies would begin again. These same movies would play on and on throughout the lonely night.

Later on that same year, I saw a headline in the *Baltimore Sun*,

"Unidentified Dancer Found Dead." I wondered if it was April, but not for long, I was busy now—I had entered, without even meaning to, the sex industry.

chapter three

June 1991
San Diego

"Her behavior is just not consistent with someone about to be married," suggested Kathryn, the pre-marital counselor.

Patrick looked smug. Here it was. Evidence. There was something flawed, something not quite right about his future wife.

"I told you," he said, shaking his head. "She goes out dancing all the time. She isn't ever home."

"I just like to dance," I said, but I knew what I did went way beyond dancing. I had wild, sordid affairs on a weekly basis. Sometimes with the same man, sometimes with a different man. I was sober from alcohol, but men were my latest six pack. Lust was my latest drug of choice.

"And she hangs out with prostitutes," Patrick lamented.

The shrink raised an eyebrow.

"Ex-prostitutes," I said.

"Why do you do that?" Kathryn asked.

I stared at a spot of lint on the carpet. "I hang out with sober people. I can't help what they used to be in their past."

"But do they all have to be hookers and homosexuals?" Patrick whined.

"We really don't have all that much in common," I said, feeling defensive. "He likes Rush Limbaugh, I don't; he's Catholic, I'm not. I guess I'm just more open minded than he is."

"Oh," she said. "I see." Then she looked back and forth between us, as if trying to sum us both up. "Are you aware that you two have different values and goals?"

I knew that we did. But I wanted to be secure and I believed that marriage would give me that.

"Her mother's suicidal, her sister's a drunk, and her father's some kind of hippie convict. And her stepfather, well he's a friggin' pedophile," Patrick said.

The counselor winced.

I just shrugged, and I thought about how this particular moment in time reminded me of a scene that had taken place when I was about fourteen. When I was growing up, my stepfather, like Patrick, was always trying to find evidence that I was a bad girl.

Kathryn was staring at me like I was some strange, exotic zoo animal. "I hate to sound repetitive, Juliet, but your behavior really is *not* consistent with a woman about to be married."

I squirmed restlessly in my seat. I was being labeled, and it made me want to run right out of the pre-marital counselor's claustrophobic office.

"So far, from what I can tell from the few meetings we have had together, you are the wild child and he wants to tame you," she said. "But you are being defiant."

I really didn't want to hear any of this.

"For example," Kathryn went on, "Patrick says that you are angry about having to annul your first marriage."

"He wants to get married in the Catholic Church, so I have to go through with it. But I don't exactly believe in all the Catholic Church believes in."

"Isn't it possible that your differences could cause conflicts down the road?"

Maybe it would, but I couldn't think about that right now—after all, I had a wedding to plan—so I didn't say anything.

Patrick scowled in my direction.

"Well, are you going to go through with the annulment?" Kathryn asked.

"Yes," I said.

"Can you two come back next week?"

I nodded, as I thought about the next man I wanted to have an affair with. I'm playing a dangerous game, you see. I'm engaged and yet I have this compulsive need to have affairs. After a while, the lies take on their own life, and soon I am living in two worlds. And for some reason I cannot stop. I always believed that I could operate with my own set of rules. It didn't matter what society did, or what was acceptable. I played the game by my own set of rules, taking from men, conning men, and lying to everyone.

I believe that the affairs, the sexual acting out, and the promiscuity are all directly related to having been incested, molested, exploited and sexualized too young and too often. Split off and removed from the innocent, precious child I had always been deep down, I acted out sexually, believing as I did that this was how to take back control of my environment.

Underneath the acting out there existed a world of painful truths that I could not admit to. Such as the fact that Patrick had an explosive temper. And that most likely this marriage really wasn't meant to be. I was running as hard and as fast as I could from both of these realities. I was having affairs, and I was justifying the affairs because I was, I told myself, just trying to get it out of my system before I got married.

I did not know then that I had a sex and love addiction. And so I was continuing to live out a pattern: going from man to man, relationship to relationship, anything but take the time to sit quietly and feel my emotions. My particular predilection also showed up as a desperate need for security. I wanted to be taken care of. I wanted prince charming to rescue me, when I was more than capable of doing all that for myself.

Because of this addiction to both love and security, I wasn't open to hearing what might be pretty good advice, or to really paying attention to what was going on. For example, Patrick's ferocious temper would not deter me from taking my vows. My family's reluctance to attend my wedding, or my friend's opinion that our wedding plans were a horrible mistake did nothing to influence my decision either. And not even the fact that I was I continuing to have affairs raised any red flags. I was going to walk down that aisle no matter what.

Patrick and I were silent as we took the elevator down to the parking lot. It seemed like the longest elevator ride I had ever been on.

"No more going out without me," he said, scowling in my direction. "And no more hanging out with people who are lower than you."

Lower than me, I thought. *He doesn't even know me at all.* I felt a sinking sensation in my chest.

"Okay," I said. But I knew deep down I was heading for trouble. Big trouble. I could never be what Patrick wanted me to be. I was an ex-hooker. I was hanging out with so called "lower people" because I was trying to learn about some of the choices we had in common. But how could I explain that? Even if I could, it wouldn't change the fact that I wasn't ready to be married.

I hadn't been ready the first time I got married, and I wasn't going to be ready this time. I was writing checks I couldn't cover, making promises I could not keep. The elevator doors opened and although we walked out together we were very separate.

That night, I pulled out my first wedding dress. Clasping the creamy, satiny folds of fabric toward my breast, I remembered . . .

***

When I was 21, I moved away from the East Coast and moved to the West Coast. I was going to be a bride for the first time. My husband-to-be would rescue me from all that had gone before. When I moved, I left behind a life that I never, ever wanted to have anything to do with again. I soon discovered that it is not that easy to just simply fly 3,000 miles to forget the past. It is always there—what I went through—and it is inside of me.

In fact, my problems started long before I climbed into that first wedding dress. My difficulties, especially around sexuality, began in my childhood home. In the home that I grew up in, a strange sexual energy abounded—it was in the every air—the very atmosphere that surrounded us, a dark cloying miasmic poison. In fact, our home should have had a "Poisonous Gas" warning label across the front door. Any female who entered our home became the latest victim of my stepfather's advances. My stepfather even hit on an aunt who came to help out after my mother made a suicide attempt.

My stepfather went into my sister's bedroom nearly every night until she was sixteen. My mother always had to make sure she was good and drunk when he advanced on her. I know that I too was sexually abused, I just can't remember very much. What I do remember is shadowy, evanescent. I can see a figure in the doorway, coming towards me. Sometimes images of a face, a face wearing horn-rimmed glasses, looms above me, larger than life. And then my conscious mind splits off, and the images recede.

Growing up with a sexual terrorist does teach coping strategies. In fact, my childhood and teenage years were excellent training ground for the aspiring hooker. First of all, just like my mother, I learned how to completely shut down. Next, I learned that men could not be trusted, and that, ultimately, the one who controlled whether or not to be sexual was the person with the power.

In my home, that person was, of course, my stepfather. My stepfather, who, with a sense of entitlement that he believed was his male birthright, took advantage of his wife, his two stepdaughters, and any other female who entered our home.

Believe me, I tried to avoid his advances—and often suffered extreme consequences. For example, one time, when I was about fourteen, when my stepfather wasn't able to have the access to me that he wanted, he tried to have me committed. I won't ever forget that day. My stepfather and mother took me to a psychiatrist's office. My stepfather took a document out of a briefcase. He explained to me that it was a copy of my journal, which apparently he had xeroxed.

"You xeroxed my journal?" I said, stunned.

"It was for your own good," the doctor said. "From reading your journal, I could see that you are exhibiting anti-social behavior. You are having sex with boys and you are smoking marijuana."

My mother looked down, avoiding eye contact with me.
"What do you think the benefits of being an in or out-patient would be?" I heard my stepfather say.

"In or out of what?" I asked, but I was pretty sure I knew.

After we were done at the shrinks, I remember sitting in Jack and the Box with my mother and I could tell by just looking at her that she was completely zoned out on Valiums. I knew right then that I was on my own. There was no way she could protect me from my stepfather. He couldn't control me and have sex with me, and that's why he wanted to put me away.

The problem was not that I was viewed as sexual. The problem was that I was not sexual with him.

The very next night, I ran away. I can't tell you how many times I went back and forth between the East Coast and the West Coast. This time when I ran away, I went to my father's house in San Francisco. I could tell right away that his wife did not appreciate my arrival. Suddenly she was faced with the mirror image of what she had been when she took him away from us. A child with sprouting, budding sexuality.

And so I began to split off inside. The vulnerable lost little girl went underground. I pretended I didn't care whether they wanted me there or not. I acted tough and cool to hide the terrified, lost little girl inside.

I grew up fending for myself and thinking that I had better know how to take care of myself, because if I didn't, nobody else would. I couldn't rely on anyone, but I did figure out pretty quickly that being young, pretty and female had its advantages.

I could use men. I could con men. My theory was it was good to be a bad girl as long as you got something in return. No one could use me if I was using them first. No one could hurt me if I was getting paid.

I think the game started when my stepfather gave my phone number to that man who took nude pictures of me. I needed money so I said sure. It was at that moment that I first began to experience the power that I possessed over men.

Soon after that I progressed from nude modeling to my one-day stint as a stripper. What happened for me is that I began to filter everything through a warped belief system. I believed that I could control men through my sexuality. My belief crystallized into an addiction and I became hooked on that control.

In my freshman year of college, I decided on Visual Performing Arts, or Theater as my course of study. That's when I met April, who, also a theater major, told me that she was going to work at the Gayety Theatre in Baltimore's red light district.

I had felt so horribly out of control that day, as I spun on the stage of that dirty floor. If only I knew then what I know now. That on that hot summer day in Baltimore, at the age of seventeen, I crossed an invisible line. My one-day career as a stripper, although short-lived, opened the door to the world of the sex industry.

Not long after that another girlfriend set up an introduction with a madam. "I think you two might have something in common," my friend explained. As it turned out, we did. The marketability of my vagina.

The madam and I sat in this coffee shop and she had proper little suit on and she just kind of sized me up, and I could tell she was pleased by what she saw. Why wouldn't she be?

I was a real find—under 18, blonde, pretty—a choice object. I wanted money for college, so I went to work for her. And that's how I worked my way through college. Turning tricks. I never *called* it that because I always thought of myself as a "call girl," and I always felt that, "well, at least I'm not out on the streets."

Making that distinction allowed me to do what I did and believe that it was something more than what it really was—a degrading, self-destructive and potentially lethal lifestyle.

In addition to the madam, I also had friends who would introduce me to these upper and middle class "gentlemen" that wanted to go out with a college coed. They would appear on my campus in their little Porsches and pick me up and take me out to some discreet apartment and have sex with me.

What happened in my life is that I developed many personas. To most people, I presented the face of a wholesome, industrious college girl. But there was another role I played equally as well—that of the whore. This facet of my fragmented personality turned tricks while living in her (my) mother's apartment. Years later I found out my mother heard all the activity from her boyfriend's apartment directly beneath ours, and wondered why I had such a sexual appetite.

I had one life as a college girl and a "good daughter," and another world as a call girl or a prostitute. Often, the two worlds I lived in collided. Drugs and alcohol helped me bridge that split between these two worlds. I made the madam give me downers, or marijuana, anything to gloss over the degrading reality of prostitution. I was becoming more and more obsessed with earning as much money as I could. Money was instant gratification—a fix.

After a while, when you have a taste for the money, you are hooked. The money becomes a fix, anesthetizing you from the truth. With money, you feel like you can conquer the world. I rationalized that money gave me control. It certainly paid the tuition and the rent. For example, on a weekend at the madam's house I could earn enough to get me through a semester at college.

There certainly were little perks about being in the life. There was this facade of excitement. You met different people, you drove around in nice cars with rich men, and you did designer drugs and wore designer clothing. I tried desperately to convince myself that I enjoyed the life, or the world of the sex industry.

As I got closer to graduating from college, my addiction to the sex industry progressed. No longer was I satisfied with having just a few clients. I wanted sugar daddies, and I wanted at least five of them.

Maybe that would be enough, I thought. *Maybe that would make the pain and the fury and the desperation go away.* But nothing ever worked. There was never enough money, or gifts, or drugs to make my feelings stop.

I often wonder why my mother didn't question where all my college tuition was coming from. How could she overlook the stream of men coming in and out of my life, or the fact that her daughter was always beautifully dressed and had her bills magically paid? I believe she did not want to know the truth. Just as she did not want to know that her two daughters were being sexually abused.

* * *

I really wished I could have left the past alone, but I couldn't. Not after what happened at my mother's house. My world was spinning out of control.

chapter four

June 1991
Baltimore

    Like I said, I really wish I could have just left the past behind me. It would have been so much . . . neater. But too much has just been swept under the rug for too long and it just isn't going to get any better for any of us women until the truth comes out.

    I was feeling pretty nervous about the wedding, and concerned about my family's silence. None of them wanted to even discuss it with me, other than to tell me I was making a mistake. I decided to pay my mother a visit and try to get her to see things my way. I didn't even tell her I was coming out, just booked a flight to Baltimore and took a shuttle from the airport to her place.

    My mother wasn't home when I arrived, but her husband William let me in. He didn't exactly look thrilled to see me, but I didn't mind.

    About an hour later, my half-brother John Jr. stopped by. He had a package for my mother. "It's from John Sr.," he said.

"What is it?" I asked.

"I don't know. I don't have anything to do with him anymore. She can read it or trash it. Have to go," he said.

"Things to do."

"Yes, of course," I said. My half-brother John Jr. had always been aloof like this, so I didn't take it personally. Actually, I don't think he has even hugged me in ten years.

I peered at the package and I knew instinctively that I would have to open it. It was from my stepfather, and it contained a book, entitled *Victims of Memory: The Shattered Lives of the Accused*. After reading the book jacket and scanning a few pages I surmised that the author believed that countless men were being wrongfully accused of perpetrating sexual abuse.

My hands shaking badly, I put the book down. Then, after a moment or two, I opened a plain white envelope and read the letter—a copy of the original—that was inside it. I knew immediately my stepfather had written it. There was that sloppy, barely coherent handwriting that I hadn't seen in years.

I began to read.

Dear Ruth,

I have tried very hard since we have been divorced in 1981 to get by. As you know, I have Attention Deficit Disorder. Earlier this year, Juliet accused me of being a child molester. She said that I molested her and that she went on to say that I molested her older sister Marie until she was sixteen.

These bizarre accusations must stop. For several months afterward, I suffered from a deep and chronic depression. Thank God I had the help of all my friends, or I don't know what I would have done. If I really did do these things, then I would have had to register as a sexual offender with the Sacramento Sheriff's office. I am willing to talk to any of you about this. Please contact me immediately.

Sincerely,

John Sr.

What was very interesting about this letter of denial is that it screamed of guilt. To me, as I read between the lines, his letter said: *"I'm guilty, and I am so obsessed with what would happen to a convicted pedophile that I know all the laws, all the possible repercussions."*

My stepfather knew all the right buzz words. He had the speech down. He was claiming to suffer from adult attention deficit disorder. He also said that he had experienced a terrible head injury, and had even suffered from a mild heart attack.

Quite skillfully, the predator had transformed himself into a victim. And my stepfather had selected the perfect book to support his victimization. The author of *Shattered Lives of the Accused* made a case for all those poor, victimized pedophiles that were being falsely accused by women who apparently had nothing better to do then go around and dredge up things that may or may not have happened. These men, the author claimed, were the innocent bystanders of a nationwide witch hunt.

Clearly, my stepfather felt that he had been set up for the same nefarious plot. *How amazing,* I thought. He had completely convinced himself of his own innocence. I put the letter down. If I hadn't just read it, I never would have believed that a letter like that could possibly exist. I had always wondered what his reaction to the letter would be. Now I knew.

In the letter, I confronted my stepfather about the many years he had sexually abused and psychologically terrorized my entire family. After I accused him, I heard nothing. I did not, at that time, want to take him to court. I just wanted him to leave us alone.

My stepfather came into my life when I was three. My mother did not have the strength to leave him until I was 21. By that time, so much damage had already been done. And yet over the years, he continued to contact my sister and I, as if nothing wrong had ever happened. Once, when I was living in San Diego, I received a bizarre phone call from him. It was a rainy, stormy evening, and I had no idea how he had gotten my phone number. Perhaps hoping I might feel sorry for him, he explained at length his difficulty in finding a job. And then he asked me if I wanted to meet him at the Japanese Bathhouse located in downtown San Diego. Horrified, I hung up on him.

I had nightmares for a week after just that one phone call. On another occasion, he had called my sister who lived in San Francisco to see if *she* wanted to join him at a bathhouse in the very seedy Tenderloin district. I guess he had a thing about the water.

Finally, I had written him a letter saying that yes, he had abused all of us, and no, I did not want him to contact my sister and I.

Obviously, the package I now held in my hands showed he hadn't given up. Indeed, his package and the enclosed letter indicated that he still wasn't quite ready to leave us alone. And it also indicated that even though my stepfather had been out of the family for many years, his evil, corrosive influence lingered on.

With the letter still clutched in my hand, I closed my eyes and remembered.

My mother had made a suicide attempt. My stepfather walked up to me in the hallway of our home in Connecticut. "I told your sister there is blood on her hands if your mother dies," he said.

I was only twelve; I had no idea what he meant. Was he trying to blame my mother's suicide attempt on my sister?

Years later, my mother told me, "I made the suicide attempts to escape his domination."

There's blood on your hands . . . .

I tried to die to escape the domination.

Blood on your hands . . . .

Adrenaline coursing through my veins, I knew I would have to act. I simply could not let my mother see this letter. It would destroy her. The past was something she simply would not, and could not discuss. I didn't want her to have to start now. I just didn't think she would be strong enough.

Just then, William, my mother's third and current husband walked in. His gaze fell immediately to the letter in my hands. "What do you have there?" he inquired.

"John Jr. brought it over. It's from John Sr. It's for Mom...I, that is, ugh—"

"What is it?" he demanded.

"It's a package, and well, there's a letter in it."

"A letter?"

"Yes. And I don't think Mother should see the letter. It would upset her too much."

He frowned in my direction. "Don't you think that's for her to decide?"

"Of course," I said. "I'll just look at it a little longer, okay?"

He shrugged and walked out of the kitchen. I took the package into the guest room and placed it on a nightstand by the bed. And then I went for a walk. After my brief walk, I headed back towards the guest room.

There, at the top of the stairs, her face shrouded in shadows, stood my mother. Even the shadows could not conceal the anger in her face. "I knew exactly where to find it," she said.

I stood frozen in place at the bottom of the stairs. "You knew where to find what?"

"You know what I'm talking about."

"No, I really don't."

"I'm talking about the letter, Juliet."

"What letter?" I stammered, as I slowly, cautiously moved up the steps. The noise from each step that I took seemed amplified.

And then, as I attempted to walk by my mother, the look she directed my way sent a chill down my spine.

"It was my letter," she said, her voice shaking with emotion as she grabbed my arm. "Why did you take my letter?"

Finally, I managed to wrench myself out of my mother's vise-like grip and move towards my room.

"Answer me," she demanded, following right behind me.

"Why did you take it?"

I turned to face her. "Because I wanted to protect you—that's why. I knew it would upset you. And I—"

"Protect me, why, because I'm getting old?"

"Mother, this has absolutely nothing to do with age, believe me," I said. "I just know how upset you get, your depression being what it is," I went on, instantly regretting my words. Family members were all well aware that you did not discuss either mother's depression, or her thirty-year pill addiction.

"I feel betrayed," she said.

"You feel what?"

"You betrayed me."

"I betrayed you—I was trying to protect you."

"I didn't ask for your protection."

"But Mom, you are suic—"

"Say it—I'm suicidal. You think I'm going to read something like that and get suicidal—is that it?"

"I just thought it would be best."

"I don't know why I have to deal with things like this at my age."

"That's just it Mom, I didn't want you to have to."

"Well that should have been my decision to make."

"I just wanted to show it to Patrick, and then I was going to send it to you."

"Why would you want to show it to him?"

"I wanted him to believe me about what a crazy person John Sr. is."

"Everybody knows he's a crazy person," my mother said angrily.

Slowly, she began moving out of the room. She stood at the top of the stairs, and she had the strangest look on her face. I had seen it before.

Once, when I was about age 14, the family had taken a summer vacation to Europe that hadn't turned out very well. My mother had made an attempt on her life. I went to visit her in a Copenhagen Mental Ward. Dressed in only a paper-thin blue robe, she peered up at me. She looked both terrified, and angry.

That same mixture of emotions—terror and anger—played on her face right now. It was hard to even look at her, so I glanced down. There, in my mother's hands, ripped into small pieces, was what used to be the letter.

"I started to put it down the toilet," my mother said. "But I stopped because I was afraid there might be a flood."

"Oh," I said.

"I don't want this letter to go out of the house."

We were now both standing at the top of the stairs. Then, my mother moved down a step. The walls behind her were lined with African masks. As a child these masks had always frightened me. The first time my stepfather had molested me, we lived in a primitive village in Africa.

My stepfather collected them, and each house we lived in, there they were. I grew to hate those masks, sensing, knowing, that there was something evil about them. There was something evil in those masks, and something evil about my mother right now.

"I wanted to show that letter to Patrick," I said.

"No," my mother said. "I'm going to burn it."

"No, mother, you must not burn that letter. It's evidence."

chapter five

"Why, mom, why did you rip it up?" I said.

"It had to be destroyed."

We both stood there, staring at the tiny pieces of paper still clutched in my mother's hands.

"You shouldn't have opened my package," she said.

"I know, I'm sorry, I just didn't want you to have to see it—I thought—"

"It doesn't matter anymore. It's time we rid ourselves of evil once and for all."

"What are you going to do?" I said.

"We're going to burn this. Every piece of paper. We're going to burn it and we're going to forget all about this, forget all about him, and never, ever mention it again."

"But—"

"No, no buts. It's over. We will never, ever mention his name again."

I followed my mother down the stairs and outside onto the front porch. She crumbled the torn up letter into a little ball.

Next, she lit the corners of the letter and after a bit the white paper became eclipsed in orange and yellow flames.

We both stood there and watched until the letter disintegrated.

"It's over now," my mother said. "He can't hurt us anymore."

I nodded at my mother as she went by me and went back into the house. I sat on the front porch and peered down at the letter. Only it wasn't a letter anymore, it was ashes and tiny black particles of soot disappearing into the summer night.

My mother thought that once she burnt the letter my stepfather wouldn't be able to hurt us anymore. Once again, we were trying to deny the impact of the past. One more time we were saying, burn it up, cover it up, pretend it didn't happen. And even though my stepfather, in the letter, had denied the sexual abuse, his words were at least a reaction to the charges I had made against him.

Something invisible had at last been brought to the surface. Or at least it had been for a brief moment in time until my mother destroyed it. *Just ignore the past,* my mother's actions told me. *And then you won't have to deal with the pain.*

I know my mother had been living this way a long, long time. She had learned to shut down so that she could survive living in the same house with the perpetrator. At first she had taken those Valiums that they prescribed to women in the sixties and early seventies. Then she mixed pills with alcohol. Finally, she started taking anti-depressants. She'd been taking various forms of anti-depressants for over thirty years. If she ever tried to go off of them, the pain was so great she had to find the next family of drugs.

I do not blame my mother for wanting to numb her feelings and forget the past. But as I sat and stared at those black ashes I felt a sense of loss. And then anger. I wanted the chance to read that letter again. I wanted to try and understand my stepfather. For even in his denial that he sexually abused us, he appeared to be crying out for help.

But my mother didn't want to deal with it anymore. She would rather breathe in this dense, poisonous silence. Because breathing in the poisonous gas, however dangerous, was at least familiar.

My mother projected her sense of betrayal onto me; after all, I had read her letter. I had exposed the truth. And now I was being cast as the bad, snooping daughter. My sister, in contrast, was the good daughter who did not reveal family secrets.

Along with my older sister, Marie, I also had two brothers. One older. One younger. Alcoholism, drug addiction, and depression ran like a swamp through my family. I had found a life raft in the twelve-step programs such as Alcoholics Anonymous, and Alanon. I had found a place where I was always welcome, a place where people would say, come in, sit down, have a cup of coffee. We understand your pain.

Unfortunately, the other adult children in my family had not found that same sense of comfort in the rooms of twelve-step meetings. Instead of joining together as a family and simply discussing the past openly, we each carried the burden of our secrets within us. And so the pain became unbearable and turned into, in my mother and sister's case, untreated alcoholism and addiction. I pondered these things, and I thought about my stepfather, and I just couldn't get past this one thought. How had one man managed to cause such long-lasting damage?

I sat outside on the front steps and watched the fireflies dance and cavort. The way I see it, we all carry the truth inside of us. Deep within us. Some things we'll admit to, others we can't. At least that's about the only conclusion that I could come to as I swatted a mosquito.

My mother had ripped up, in essence, my stepfather's confession. In the distance on that hot, sultry Baltimore night, a siren wailed. Someone had made a false move. Someone had committed a crime. And perhaps there would be some form of justice. *Justice,* I thought, as I hugged my knees to my chest. I wasn't so sure about justice. It seemed to me that any attempts at justice had just gone up in smoke.

The next day, my mother drove me to Baltimore Washington airport. Just as she had done so many times while I was growing up, my mother got us lost. In her defense, it is true that we were constantly moving back then, and so it is fairly understandable that she would lose her sense of direction more often than not. Nevertheless, I found my mother's inability to get us where we needed to be absolutely terrifying. Anyway, when she did finally manage to locate the airport, she dropped me off without even giving me a goodbye hug. As I watched her drive off I knew that our relationship had changed forever.

"And to your right is the Grand Canyon," the pilot droned, interrupting me from that limbo land between being awake and sleeping.

I peered out of the airplane window at the geological splendor below me. As I studied the deep chasms and rising crests of the Grand Canyon, I thought about distances. In particular, the psychological distances between my family members. We were all divided from each other, each isolated in our own world of personal pain. And for the most part, the cause of our family's estrangement had to do with my stepfather. One more time I wondered how one person could have such an impact. It just didn't make sense.

And so as the plane flew over the Grand Canyon, I knew something that I hadn't known before my brief visit home. My mother could not stand the truth and believed admitting the truth would completely destroy her. In contrast, I believed that it was only through fully examining and understanding the impact of the past that I could truly live my current life. As a result of the differing viewpoints my mother and I shared, I had the feeling I wouldn't hear from my mother for a long time.

And sure enough, after I got home, I didn't hear from my mother for over a month. She had sent some pictures of our visit. I couldn't help but notice that, on the envelope, she had used my first name along with my stepfather's last name, which I had banished some twenty years earlier.

I couldn't stand the silence, and I finally called.

"I've been so angry at you," my mother said.

"At me?"

"Yes. At your betrayal—and don't try to deny it."

There it was. I betrayed her. I was trying to protect her from the truth, because I knew she would be devastated by it. Since I was the one who opened the letter, since I was in essence the messenger, I had become the target of my mother's rage.

chapter six

July 1991
San Francisco

After visiting with my mother on the East coast, I really needed to talk to my sister Marie. I wanted to talk to her about the letter. I needed to know if it really was true. About the sexual abuse and all. I mean, maybe it really was like in that book, *Victims of Memory, The Shattered Lives of the Accused*. Maybe, like the women in the book, we were just confused, misguided. Maybe we'd made up what had happened to us in the past, and our memories were a sort of free-floating fiction.

I hopped on a plane to San Francisco. Just a few hours later the driver of an airport van dropped me off at my sister's place located in a small neighborhood called the Sunset District. I pressed the doorbell under my sister's mailbox and the front door lock was released. I made my way upstairs.

"I'm so glad you're here," my sister said warmly. "I've missed you."

"I've missed you too," I said, giving my sister a big hug.

"Where's your son?"

"Tommy is sleeping, would you like to see him?"

I nodded, and followed her to his room. "He's so cute," I whispered, so as not to wake Tommy. "I'm so happy for you—this is what you've always wanted."

"*He's* what I've always wanted," Marie said frankly. "I don't know about everything else."

As we were leaving Tommy's room, I smelt it—the unmistakable odor of alcohol. For over ten years, my sister had been in the chronic stages of alcoholism.

Reluctantly, I put the question to her. "Have you been drinking, Marie?"

"I knew you were going to ask that," she replied defensively.

"So…is that a yes?"

"Stop looking at me like that!"

"Oh, Marie, why?"

"Reasons to drink? The list is endless, but don't start with me about that, or going to AA meetings. This is complicated."

"It always is."

"I can't go to AA meetings because I'm a prisoner here. You need to know that right away. So don't even bother to ask me to go meetings, because my husband won't let me."

"Sure, okay," I agreed, and I put my bags down in the spare room. There, in the corner of the room, was the same couch that I called home when I was sixteen years old.

* * *

1975
San Francisco

When I was sixteen and Marie was 21, I had run away one more time and I was living on my sister's couch. My sister was a Women's Studies major at San Francisco State, and the second wave of the women's movement was well underway.

One day, my sister Marie handed me a book about women's anatomy. She opened up the book and handed it to me. "Here," she said. "This is a picture of a vagina. This is what it looks like both on the inside and the outside of your body."

"I don't want to look at...*that*," I said resolutely, pushing the offensive book away.

The V word flickered through my mind like a cheap neon sign that turns on and off in a corner window of a dimly lit dive bar. *Vagina. Vagina.* I wasn't sure if I had ever heard the word spoken out loud before. It was something you weren't supposed to say. It was part of the female anatomy, and so it was shameful, dark, and ugly.

"Just look at it, Juliet," my sister insisted.

Warily, I looked at the picture she held out to me. The picture had arrows pointing to specific areas, like the clitoris. "What's a clitoris?" I asked.

"It's the woman's pleasure center. In my women's consciousness raising group we have been learning about discovering the power of the clitoris. The first thing you have to be able to do is find it. So what you do is use a hand-held mirror, and hold it down there so you can see it."

"You're crazy," I said.

I had never heard of a clitoris let alone look at one, especially my own. For some reason I was terrified of my sexual body. It was perplexing that despite my fear and terror about sex I was so promiscuous. And it was equally perplexing that despite my promiscuity I knew nothing about my sexual anatomy.

"No, I'm not crazy," Marie insisted. "You'll see. Your clitoris is beautiful, and it will be liberating for you to find it." Then my older sister handed me a large mirror. "Go in my room and look for it."

I couldn't believe that she wanted me to go look at a part of my body that scared me like it did. But I could tell I didn't have a choice, and so, reluctantly, mirror in hand, I locked myself in her room. It took me a while to muster up enough courage to begin my investigation. After all, I had never seen that part of my body before. As I spread my legs apart, I felt like a complete idiot. Waves of shame and embarrassment washed over me, but still I continued on my quest, eventually discovering the buried treasure. There, tucked beneath the pink folds was a little galaxy I had never known existed. Absolutely horrified, I threw the mirror down.

What happened to me, I wondered. *Why was I numb and frozen in that area? Why couldn't I even say the word "vagina?"*

At sixteen, I really did not want to believe bad things had happened. How could it be true? The evil my sister spoke about. My stepfather touching us like she said he did.

I decided that she was just too sensitive, and maybe just a little crazy.

That was what they tried to tell us when we were growing up—that there was something wrong with Marie. I'm pretty sure it was my stepfather who wanted us all to believe that. Especially since Marie used to complain about him wanting to french kiss her and all. I'm just trying to show her my affection, he would protest to my mother, who would then yell at us girls that we weren't allowing John Sr. to be our father.

Of course, as a young girl, I possessed neither the words nor the awareness to tell Mom that, in general, french kissing is not a part of being a dad. Anyway, at the wise old age of sixteen, I couldn't believe anything had happened to my sister, because if it had happened to her, then maybe it could have happened to me. I hid behind a facade of coolness and toughness. From that perspective, it was easier to believe that nothing had ever been as bad as she said it was—it just couldn't have been.

I was beginning to learn the art of disassociation.

Wearing my denial and my anger like a cloak, I walked the streets of San Francisco and wondered where I would live and why my own father didn't want me to stay with him. I guess I was what you would call a throwaway kid. Disposable.

I wanted to see if I could get my father to change his mind about me living with him. I knew my days of living on Marie's couch were numbered, so I went to see my post-beatnik, hippie, part-time convict father in the Haight-Ashbury. I begged him to let me stay there again. *Let me come home, father, please.*

His Japanese wife looked at me with contempt. I knew what she was thinking. I was sixteen—didn't I know how to take care of myself? I was expected to be an adult so that it would be convenient for them. I could drink with them, but I could not be a child with needs and wants.

She didn't want me there, and because she didn't want me there, my father didn't want me either. I told myself it was just fine that way, besides I didn't need them anyway. I didn't need anyone. Feeling something hard forming around my heart, I caught the 7-Haight downtown to Market Street.

On the bus that cold, foggy San Francisco morning, I remember peering over someone's newspaper and reading the headlines: HEIRESS KIDNAPPED! Patty Hearst had been kidnapped. Strangely enough, I felt envious. At least someone wanted her enough to steal her. Maybe if I was kidnapped my father would care about me.

Since my father didn't want to take care of me, I had to find another job. And fast. I always found it ironic that my father was so insistent on me having a job, since *he* never had one. I had never known him to have a job—other than the ones provided by the California Department of Corrections.

I went to live in some speed freak's basement who had hired me to take care of her three kids so that she could pull all-nighters at the donut shop. I'll never forget that basement. It was dark and damp and the shadows freaked me out. To cope, I started swallowing black beauties like candy. Her boyfriend started coming on to me, molesting me. It never occurred to me that what he was doing was against the law. I didn't like it, but my innocence had already been stolen. I just thought that's what men did, they took what they wanted, and in return, they would give me something so that I would feel less afraid, something that warmed up that cold darkness scratching at my heart.

When I was living down in San Francisco, just a few years after the flower children days, there were many not-so-young anymore hippies who wanted to teach me all about "free love," or sex with minors, or girls who were too stoned to really know what was happening to them. Perhaps now it would be called date rape, instead of "free love."

Once, Mary, the speed freak, called the cop on her so-called boyfriend, when she found out he was having sex with both of us. I remember when the cops came to the door; they looked at me, and, incredulous, asked, "Aren't you a little young to be on your own?"

I just smiled and went down in the basement and told myself that those cops were crazy. I *wasn't* too young to be on my own! I was free! I had a job, and I had a place to live. I didn't need anyone to take care of me. But that cop's reaction had jarred my fantasy world, and my new home suddenly looked as if it might be suitable only for small rodents.

That night I kept on as many lights as I could in a desperate attempt to shut out the darkness and shadows that shape-shifted all around me. The terror I felt never really subsided, and the day after I graduated from my alternative high school, where I had majored in backpacking and getting high, I took off.

And then, a week later, maybe a month, it was hard to say back then, I hopped on another Greyhound bus. Eating Cheetos and reading *True Confessions* magazines, anger and confusion swirled in my gut. I was always on the move, the terror of being a teenager in America nipping at my heels. No matter where I went, whether by Greyhound bus, train or plane, I never found the comfort I so desperately sought.

The next stop on my journey was Wilbur Hot Springs in Napa Valley. It was one of those holistic health new age aren't we-organic type places. I was hired to be a maid and to baby-sit the owner's three-year old daughter. But my employment was cut short when they insisted that I participate in their Gestalt therapy treatment program. What this basically meant is that they wanted me to work for free, and while I was at it, perform sexual favors for the doctor, who also happened to be the owner.

When I refused to participate in their "program" I was asked to leave. I was on the move again. I wasn't afraid; I knew how to survive, after all I had my tough girl act well in place. I knew how to pull down that mask that said, "I may look young but you better treat me like I'm an adult." This defiance kept me alive for many years. But it also made me feel horribly alone. At times, I felt as if I was falling down a long, endless tunnel and I knew there would be no one to catch me at the other end. On a constant basis I experienced an indescribable fear that reverberated down to my very core.

I crisscrossed back and forth from San Francisco to Baltimore, believing that as soon as I got to wherever I was running to my parents would rush towards me with open arms and tell me how much they wanted me in their lives. But it never turned out that way.

On another occasion, still in my teens, my father gave me five weeks to live with him. I had to get a job by that time, or I was out. I was so scared- what would I do-where would I live?

Combing the streets of downtown San Francisco, the old men hooted at me, chicken hawking they call it..."Hey little girl, you lost? Come and sit on daddy's lap."

I just kept walking. Something always kept me safe, protected, despite the dangerous circumstances I often found myself in.

Somehow, I managed to find a job at a beauty salon. By that time, however, Jake, my father, had already gotten himself locked up. Chino, I think it was, or maybe it was Tracey. He'd been in so many state prisons it was hard to keep up with the names. So even though I had the job, one more time, I had to leave.

I drifted up and down the coast of Northern California, staying with whoever would have me, which was, in most cases, males with selfish motives. Finally, after weeks of tearful phone calls to my mother back in Maryland, there was some good news. I could come back home. My stepfather had changed his mind about me. Unfortunately, it turned out that just like the strangers who had provided me with temporary shelter, my stepfather also had ulterior motives.

He had decided he wanted me to attend the university where he was a distinguished college professor of human sexuality. I was even asked to attend several weekend-long seminars on the various aspects of sexuality. There, and at the university, he took full advantage of the status a pretty stepdaughter granted him. In both institutions, whether it was during seminars or at the university, my stepfather delighted in engaging me, in groups of equally fascinated guests, about matters of a sexual nature. Had I had sex with other girls, he would ask, and if so, how often, and so on and so forth.

While this might have been an appropriate exchange with a grown up, it was not with his under-age stepdaughter. But I hadn't figured that out yet. It was, however, pretty clear to me that sex, in our home, was all-

powerful and larger than life.

My mother and stepfather let me live with them a short time, but then, when I would not act like his surrogate girlfriend, I was asked to leave. At that point, nothing mattered. I had no boundaries and no emotions other than desperation. Wholeness and personal dignity were foreign concepts to me I was ready. I was a perfect homegrown candidate for prostitution.

chapter seven

July 1991
San Francisco

And now, all these years later, I wanted to know why I had made the choices I made. And I wanted to understand how what happened to us as girls, when we were sexually abused, had contributed to the choices I made both in the past and in my present.

My sister had always been a bridge I could count on, her memories and insights connecting me to my own truth.

"I'm getting fat, unlike you, Miss Thin and Perfect one." Marie drifted off to a mirror to look at herself. "You were always the pretty one."

"Come on Marie, you're pretty too."

"No, I'm not. Not according to my husband. He thinks I'm an ugly cow. Besides, I'm bruised, everywhere."

"He hits you?" I said, shocked. What had happened to my feminist sister?

"I told you," Marie said, "I'm a prisoner here."

"I'm sorry," I said. "Will he…will he let you come to the wedding? You are coming to the wedding aren't you?"

She peered at me. "You always got the husbands didn't you, and the beautiful weddings, and the money. And everybody always said, 'Juliet's so pretty; she's the pretty one.'"

"Do we have to get into all this right now?" I said. "I wanted to talk about my wedding. I'd like you to be a bridesmaid."

"You don't seem to understand. I can't go to your wedding."

"Because of your husband?"

"That isn't all of it," Marie admitted.

"What is it then?"

"Mother made me promise I wouldn't go."

My heart started pounding.

"She said, 'promise me, promise me that you won't go, Momma won't like it if you go,' that's what she said."

"She didn't really say that—did she?" I watched my sister nodding that yes, she really had said that. An all-too familiar curtain of hurt descended just then. All my life I had felt that my mother and sister's intense, love-hate relationship left me out in the cold. I always felt invisible.

Why had I become the enemy? Why was I the scorned daughter? I was walking through a mystery that I felt ill equipped to solve. "What is it with you two?" I asked, desperate to understand why my own mother would say such a thing.

"She thinks you're rushing into this. She thinks you're getting married for the wrong reasons. She thinks you're getting married for the same reason that you did the first time—for security."

"Why is she so judgmental when it comes down to me getting married?"

"She doesn't want us to make the same mistakes she did, I guess. And if you're going to be asking me all these questions, then

I need another drink."

I followed her into the kitchen. She took a bottle of vodka out of the fridge and poured it into a glass. She then poured orange juice into that. I let her drink that drink for a while, knowing full well that she would tell me more if she was a bit high.

"Look, Marie," I said cautiously. "There's something I need to tell you. Something happened at Mom's. A package came for her, and I opened it...It was from John Sr. I know I shouldn't have opened it—but I did. And once I read the letter he wrote I knew it would destroy her if she read it."

"We all try so hard to protect her, don't we?" Marie said.

"Did you try and protect her too?" I asked.

"Yeah, I protected her; I was practically her mother, for chrissakes. Hell, I even became his surrogate wife so that he would leave her alone."

"It happened then—didn't it? He did sexually abuse us, didn't he?"

"You're kidding right?"

I shook my head, embarrassed by my own ignorance. "No, I'm not."

"Of course he did," said Marie. "You mean you really don't know? Don't you remember?"

"That's the problem. I don't."

"It's the strangest thing," my sister said, her tone bitter. "You never remember a damn thing. In a way, I envy you. But right now, I need another drink."

"Don't you think you should pace yourself?"

"I'm getting another drink," she snapped back at me.
I followed her once more into the kitchen and watched as she poured another drink. We returned to the living room.

"Remember when I wrote to John Sr. and confronted him about the sexual abuse?"

Marie nodded.

"He denies that anything ever happened," I continued, watching her reaction carefully. She grimaced. "He said the allegations were bizarre and sent him into a deep depression."

Marie slammed her glass down so hard I was afraid it would break. Vodka splattered all over her. "Well, isn't that just too damn bad."

I got up and found something to wipe up the mess. "I'm sorry. I didn't mean to upset you."

Her hand trembled as she picked up her drink and drank what hadn't spilled. "It's not your fault. It just seems like he thinks we're all supposed to feel sorry for him." On automatic, she rose and walked over to the fridge and retrieved the bottle. This time she brought it with her and placed it back down next to her glass. "Don't you see, that letter—his denial—it was really a confession."

"I thought the same thing," I said.

"Where is the letter?"

I paused, and then said, "It's gone."

"What do you mean it's gone?"

"Mother ripped it up and then she burned it."

A shrewd look flickered across her face. "Destroying the evidence."

I nodded. "He sent a book too."

"What book?"

"*Victims of Memory: The Shattered Lives of the Accused.*"

"You have to be kidding me," she said, disgusted.

"That was the name of the book," I confirmed.

"Do you have it?" Marie asked.

"I ripped it up."

"You ripped up a book?"

"I was angry."

"Maybe you and mom should just start a paper-shredding

company," Marie said, emitting a strange, cackling laugh that I attributed more to the alcohol than anything else.

Besides, I knew what she was thinking. She thought that I was doing a tap dance with the facts. She thought I was just like our mother. In other words, destroying the book was no different from destroying the letter. And damn it, maybe she was right. Deep down, I knew that none of us would be free until we could openly face up to all that had happened.

"So, you think his saying nothing ever happened was really a confession?" I said.

"Of course it is," Marie said.

"Tell me again what happened," I said. "Tell me what he used to do to you."

She sighed deeply. Her body language indicated she was going there, to the scene of the crime. She looked sad, and, wincing slightly, she began to tell me what happened. "He came into my room nearly every night until I was sixteen years old."

"Why did it stop when you were sixteen?"

"I told a family therapist and then he stopped," Marie said.

"What exactly did he do to you?" I said.

"He always waited until mom was asleep—or passed out, whichever came first. Then, I'd hear him coming towards my room. I'd watch the door opening." She paused, remembering. "The light coming from the hallway always seemed blinding, and in all that light, I could never see his eyes. His silhouette against all that light always seemed so huge. The last thing he'd always do before he came in my room was look behind him, to make sure no one was watching."

"And then," I said, not sure if I really wanted to hear what was coming.

"Then he'd start up his little ritual."

"His ritual?"

"He'd start by giving me all these warnings. Like if I told anybody, I would be in big, big trouble. Or I had been a bad girl and he needed to teach me a lesson. Then he'd rub his fat, *filthy*, disgusting hands all up and down my body. He touched me in places that no child should ever be touched."

"Oh Marie, I'm so sorry you had to go through all that."

"Well then be just as sorry for yourself, because he did the same things to you, you just don't remember it."

"I wish I could remember, I really do."

"No, it's better that you don't."

"Did he ever—"

"No—he never did that—never penetrated me," Marie said. "He took it right to the edge, right to the limit of his sick, twisted passions. And then he would stop. Each time it happened I prayed it would be the last. But it never was."

"How did you get through it?" I said.

"Mostly I just pretended that it wasn't happening. As soon as he came into the room, I would float above myself. Then, I'd make up all kinds of stories."

How sad that my sister's fertile, rich imagination, may have, in part, been developed out of necessity. To survive.

chapter eight

I really shouldn't have gone down to the liquor store to pick up my sister another bottle of vodka, since I'm a recovering alcoholic and all. But since I wanted the information to continue flowing, I went. I walked through San Francisco's Sunset district, a small neighborhood flanked by the Golden Gate Park. My sister had lived in this neighborhood for many years; in fact, we used to drink together in many of the local bars.

As I strolled, I glanced into some of these establishments. They looked pretty much the same, and I could have sworn I recognized some of the patrons. There were lots of ghosts for me in this city…I could feel them lurking.

* * *

Sometime in The Seventies
San Francisco

My career as a runaway began at the age of fourteen, when in the dead of the night, I had hitched a ride to the airport so that I could fly to California where my father lived. Since it was one of the brief periods in his criminal career that he wasn't locked up, I knew I had to act quickly. If I waited too long, he might be incarcerated by the time I got there. Besides, I felt I would be safer with him than with my molesting stepfather, who had tried to put me into a home for bad girls, or "antisocial" teens.

But my father was busy drinking with his alcoholic wife. Besides, his wife made it clear that she didn't want any competition for his attention, especially since he was hardly around. And so I moved on, and I continued to do so for the duration of my teen years.

I lived on Greyhound buses. Often, it was the only place I felt safe. En route, to the next small town, where this time things would be different. There was something so comforting about the quiet, monotonous anonymity of a Greyhound bus. Mile after mile, with nothing to do but read confessional magazines, eat junk food, and watch the strange parade of people getting on and off the bus. On each Greyhound, at least for the duration of the bus ride, I had a temporary home.

During my years on the road, one thing my father did give me was an old, beat-up suitcase. I traveled back and forth between small towns up and down the California coast, carrying the same tired old bag. The suitcase made me a target. It gave off the distinct impression of abandonment and neglect. I stood in a bus station, looking for my father.

* * *

A couple of years had gone by since the first time I ran away, and now I'm sixteen, almost seventeen. Vultures who preyed off the young lurched around me, their noses opening up to the scent of fresh meat on the line. The latch on my suitcase had given way. My meager belongings scattered across the dirty floor. Included in the chaos were photographs—the nude photographs my stepfather's friend had taken of me.

"Nice picture," a stranger said. He was a Moonie; I could tell by his smile, which reminded me of the Joker in the Batman Cartoon.

"Thanks," I said, scrambling to whisk the pictures out of sight.

The Moonie magically produced a plastic bag for all my things. He then told me about a beautiful farm in Mendocino. "You will be a part of a big family," he explained.

But I knew his game. He was looking for prospects. I'd seen pictures of their mass weddings in *Life* magazine. Even though I knew the Moonies were a cult, for a split second going with him didn't seem like such a bad idea. And so I took his number down, just in case nothing else worked out for me.

Once again, as I had already done several times, I scanned through the bus station and tried to catch a glimpse of my father's face. My heart was beating fast with anticipation. Everything would be all right this time, I just knew it. Any minute he would rush up to me and give me a bear hug. Then he would—

"So you'll call tonight, right?" the Moonie said.

"Yeah sure," I said, and turned my back to him. Just then, I could have sworn I saw my father. *It simply had to be him.* Then, it seemed like I went into a trance. I had to sit down on a bench since I felt a little dizzy. I closed my eyes and the Greyhound bus station wasn't there for a minute, and instead, all I could see was this one special moment I had shared with my father. He told me he loved me. Sure, he was drunk when he said it, but he meant it. We were happy and I was safe and I belonged.

Then, someone nudged me on the shoulder. "Hey girl—you all right?"

"Daddy?" I said hopefully, opening my eyes. But it wasn't daddy.

"Why don't you come with me to Mendocino now," persisted the Moonie guy. "We have a bed for you. I just called them. Everyone wants to meet you."

"Who wants to meet me?" I said, confused for a moment.

"All the loving members of your new family."

"Look, my father's going to be here soon."

My new friend looked around. "What's he look like?"

I wasn't sure how to describe my dad, so I didn't say anything, hoping that if I just ignored him he would leave me alone. Then, finally, after standing there side by side for nearly an hour with the cult member who wanted to be my new dad, I had to admit to myself that my father wasn't coming.

Feeling suddenly much older than my sixteen years, I picked up my plastic bag and what was left of my suitcase, and headed out towards downtown San Francisco. I would have to take a bus to my father's place in the Haight-Ashbury. My stomach was growling. A swarthy-faced Greek offered me a job at a sandwich shop. At least if I worked there, I wouldn't be hungry. But something about the way he was leering at me made me nervous, so I kept moving, my bags growing heavier and heavier.

On Front Street, old derelicts sprawled on the concrete steps of a condemned building whistled and hooted at me. I quickened my pace and looked straight ahead. Turning on Broadway Street, neon signs flashed the theme of San Francisco's red light district.

LIVE NUDE GIRLS . . . ACTION . . . COME ON IN . . . RIGHT BEFORE YOUR EYES WE'VE GOT TOPLESS CUTIES . . . BAD GIRLS GALORE . . .

In this neon-ridden fantasyland of theaters named the Pussycat, Girly Parlor, or Pure Platinum, I was an immediate attraction. "Hey there baby," called out an obese black man. "Want an audition?"

"Not from you," I muttered. A stringy-haired creature of questionable gender walked by and winked. It wore a skirt, but the coarse dark hair poking through fishnet stockings seemed decidedly masculine. A girl about my age leaned provocatively over a limousine; dark tinted windows silently floated open. She persuaded the elderly man of her assets in the marketplace, and then got in.

Distracted by my reflection in a carnival-like mirror next to a Polish hotdog stand, I stood there, transfixed by what I saw: a scared, wide-eyed little girl. I twisted my ankle rushing away from the image.

"Damn," I said out loud.

Just then, a man walked by, smiling at me as he passed. "Hey there pretty girl, can I buy you a cup of coffee?"

I kept walking, doing my best to ignore him.

"Can I help you with your suitcase?" he asked, and tugged at it as if he was trying to take it from me.

I yanked my suitcase away from him. "Leave me alone!"

"Let me ask you something, when's the last time you ate something?"

"I said leave me alone," I snapped at him.

"Your loss, baby. Suit yourself."

I kept moving. Only in moving was I safe.

I made it to my father's place, and within a week he started in on me about finding a job. I often started my job hunt search by hanging out in the Golden Gate Park. As I walked through the rose garden, I felt so alone. A black man approached me. He asked me if I wanted a job doing gardening.

Back then, I didn't know that you weren't supposed to talk to strangers. I had never been taught that. One day, instead of working, the stranger wanted to watch me take a bath. Since I had no boundaries around my sexuality, I said yes. I recall that on another occasion he took me to a bathhouse where he fondled and molested me.

When I quit one day, my father was furious. I had no words to explain what had really happened to me, or why I wanted to quit. "But he was such a nice man," my father insisted.

Yeah, a nice man. A nice man who had sexually molested, harassed and victimized a minor. Other names of crimes come to mind, having more to do with my father than the man who molested me. Terms like child endangerment and failure to provide parental supervision.

And there were so many other moments when my very life was at stake. Once, still no more than sixteen, I was with another girl, backpacking along the coast. Alone. Two girls. Some guy picked us up and I remember that my friend watched, horrified, as he fondled my breasts.

"I wish I could cut these off and take them with me," the stranger said.

Now, yes, there was something horribly wrong with events like that. But I felt powerless. I did not know that I had the right to set a sexual boundary. Besides, in the seventies, people weren't talking about sexual boundaries. Not until the more chaste, AIDS-conscious 90's did such awareness come into fruition.

Anyway, in my teens, and until I took control (so I mistakenly thought) as a teenage prostitute, I just thought that whatever a man wanted to do with me he could do, and I never thought to question it. I became the bad girl, the slut, because that was what was expected of me. *My stepfather had trained me well.*

* * *

July 1991
San Francisco

Everywhere I went, I thought, as I turned a corner in my sister's neighborhood, I had been prey. The hunted. As I clutched my sister's bottle of vodka to my chest, I felt a deep sense of gratitude that I had made it out of those years alive. I had survived both family and cultural incest.

In the process of healing from being both an incest survivor and a prostituted woman, I re-claim my sexual identity when I tell the truth about how I became split from myself. How the wounded little girl went underground and how I developed into the badgirl/whore to protect her. Sure, it would be easier to pretend nothing happened. But that would be a crime. More of a crime than you can possibly imagine.

When most people think of mysteries, they think of Jessica Fletcher in the television series *Murder She Wrote*. Five minutes before the show ends she figures out the connection between a series of clues and solves the case.

But what about the crimes that no one sees, the crimes that go on behind closed doors? These crimes can go on for years, even decades. There may not be blood at the crime scene, and so the perpetrator goes undetected. One day the victim wakes up from a bad dream. In this nightmare, perhaps the woman sees the blurry outline of a perpetrator. Only it turns out it wasn't a dream. That is what happened to me.

I'm still trying to wake up from the dream. I'm still trying to get out of that basement.

When my stepfather sexually abused my sister and I, he committed murder. A little death of the psyche. A death of innocence. By the time my sister left home at the age of nineteen she was almost catatonic. And today, her life is in danger. Grave danger. Either her alcoholism or the domestic violence may kill her. And it may not happen this year. Or even the next. And maybe she will be alive physically, but there will really only be a shell of a person left.

Incest, just like prostitution, has an aftermath.

And my mother? My mother is a drug addict. She won't admit this—she'll never have to. After all, her little pills are a form of slow suicide. Slow, socially acceptable suicide. My mother's preoccupation with death is just one of our family's dirty little secrets.

My point is this: one man's poison can be slow and yet still very lethal. My stepfather's malevolence stretches across a lifetime. A vast network of family denial, lies, and secrets blanket the crime. He killed my mother's spirit off at about, say, age thirty. Handed her some pills, insulted and demeaned her on a constant basis, and then turned around and sexually molested her two teenaged stepdaughters.

No big deal. Happens all the time. It's not like he raped us or anything. And so I had always tried to just shut it out, minimize the damage. The only problem with that is this: the unexamined life gets repeated, over and over again in endless loops.

For most of my life, I tried to pretend that only my sister had been abused. And then my own memories started floating to the surface.

"For chrissakes," my sister sputtered. "What the hell took you so long?"

Marie grabbed the bottle out of my hand. After a few moments, when she had her alcohol level up to par, she began to talk.

"He was always trying to control you. He wanted to have his way with you. But there was something in you that fought him. Once you even hit him."

"I did?"

"Here we go again," she said, shaking her head.

"Do you think I like not remembering anything?" I paused, and said, "I *do* remember he was always following us around with a camera. I guess I never thought about it until now, but some of the pictures he took of us really weren't that innocent, were they?"

My sister shook her head, after a while, she said, "He used to dress us up in mother's negligees and we would dance for him. And then there were all the pictures he took of us in the bathtub."

"Yeah, he had some kind of a weird thing about us in the bathtub, didn't he?" I frowned, feeling disgusted by the memories. "I have this picture of me he took when I was about three. I only had underwear on. For years, I put that picture on the wall wherever I went. But then when I started to get more aware of things, the picture made me very nervous. I haven't put it back on the wall since."

I suppose you could speculate that my stepfather's obsession with cameras was purely innocent. But around him, I had the same sensation as when I walked in that bad part of town in San Francisco. I was prey, a creature he sexualized and objectified. And he made every female who came near him feel that way. My sister and I, as well as any other woman that came into the house, were immediately scrutinized for sexual potential.

"Remember when Mom made that suicide attempt and Aunt Victoria flew out from California to help us?" I asked. My sister nodded. "Well, a few years ago I spoke with her and she told me how uncomfortable our stepfather made her feel. Here our Mother had just tried to kill herself and he's in there hitting on her sister."

"So that was why she kept taking off, even though Mom needed her help," Marie commented.

"I can't say I blame her. And then there was the time he gave my name to a man who took nude pictures of me," I said, remembering.

"I didn't know that."

"His hands were shaking when he took the pictures."

"That's sexual abuse, you know. You were underage. He was our stepfather, supposedly our caregiver—someone we were supposed to trust. It was wrong for him to set that up."

"Yeah, I know. Sometimes I keep thinking about Africa. About when we lived in Africa, in that primitive village. And I wonder if he deliberately isolated all of us, so that we were…"

"Accessible?" Marie said.

"Yes," I said. "Something happened in Africa. I remember complaining to Mom about some rash I had down there. I remember our stepfather John Sr. was there. Something was wrong…that's all I can remember."

"Yes, I remember that too, Juliet. You were five; I was ten. I remember thinking there was something wrong with his, well, his involvement, and fascination with your…rash." She looked down, avoiding my eyes. "That should have just been something Mom handled. She was just always so out of it."

I stared at my sister's bottle and it was beginning to look intriguing. I had never noticed such intricate designs on a label before. It wasn't a good sign that all of a sudden I was so interested.

"He used to French kiss me," she said.

Now the label on the bottle was fascinating beyond belief. Perhaps, I thought, perhaps I should rip it off and really study it. I hadn't peeled a label off a bottle in a long, long time. In my beer drinking days, label peeling had been one of my favorite pastimes.

Or, better yet, to hell with all that, I thought. *Maybe I needed to forget about the label and take a drink of what was inside of the bottle.*

"You look like you're going to be sick," Marie said.

"He stuck his tongue down your throat?" I said.

"Yes, he did. Whenever he got the chance."

I stopped looking at her bottle and looked instead into her

eyes. My sister's eyes. Those eyes that had always seen so much. Too much.

"You look upset, Juliet," my sister said, gently. "Maybe we can talk about this more later."

"No, it's okay. I want to talk about it now. It's just that, well, why did all the bad stuff have to happen to you?"

"It didn't just happen to me. You just can't remember as much as I do."

"I know," I admitted, shaking my head. "I wish I could remember something more…more than just fragments."

"You were sexually abused," Marie said. "That's all you need to remember."

"But I want to remember more," I said emphatically. "I need to remember more. I am so tired of getting so close to a memory—so close—so close that I can almost touch it, only to have it disappear, and then I start thinking I'm just making the whole thing up."

"Well you didn't," Marie said with conviction.

"One time, I was getting a massage, and all of a sudden, I pictured John Sr.'s face hovering over me. He looked so big. He was wearing those dark horn-rimmed glasses."

"He used to wear glasses like that."

"I figured it didn't mean anything, and so I shoved the memory away," I said.

"It's strange," Marie said. "Those damn things we say didn't happen change the rest of our lives."

"So, do you think something really happened to me?"

Marie nodded. "Of course it did, Juliet. I think getting that massage triggered a memory you had buried for years."

"But what can we do about it?" I said. "Don't you think we should report him?"

"What good would that do?" Marie said. "It would just upset everyone, especially mom. We've got to leave it alone."

"Leave it alone, yeah, right," I said, beginning to pace the room. "It seems like that's what we've done our whole lives. Just try and forget about what he did to us. But how can we when what happened then is still happening to both of us now?"

"What are you talking about?"

"We're both in abusive relationships, and you're still drinking," I said.

"I'm drinking because of the abuse," she said. "It's the only way I can cope."

"You said before you are a prisoner here, is that true Marie?"

"Of course it's true. *I'm* a prisoner, but *you* don't have to be. You don't have to get married again. You guys aren't right for each other. He's always putting you down. It'll get worse, you know."

"What will get worse?"

"Patrick's temper. Mark my words."

"It'll get better when I'm married."

"If you say so, but I think you might end up regretting it."

"I'm *going* to go through with this. I'm getting married," I said. "And I'd like you to be there for me."

"I can't—I just can't," Marie said. "Oh, there goes the baby, and my husband will be here soon, so can we drop this for now?"

"That's all we ever do. We drop it; pretend it never happened. I think we should try and press charges. Take him to court."

"No—" Marie said firmly. "We can't do that to Mom—she would never forgive us. It would be too painful for her. We have to…"

"Protect her."

She nodded, and squeezed her glass so tightly that her knuckles turned white and for the second time in less than an hour I was afraid it would break into a million pieces.

Later that evening, needing to clear my head and sort through the thoughts and emotions swirling within, I took a walk through my old neighborhood. A damp, lonely, murkiness shrouded the Haight-Ashbury. I walked past the white Victorian home on the corner of Page and Schrader. I had lived here for a few years with my father and his wife.

* * *

When my stepfather tried to have me committed, I ran here, to the Haight-Ashbury. I was out of control, my stepfather had said. A sexual, bad girl who needed to be punished. I believe it's called blaming the victim. Since I wouldn't be his whore, I was a bad girl who needed "help." Instead, I ran, here…to San Francisco.

I thought I would be welcomed, but I wasn't. My father and his wife were drunks who didn't want the responsibility of a teenage daughter. Perhaps I was a threat to her. I was a throwaway kid…disposable. And so I ran away again, and I didn't stop running.

I turned up Page Street and cut over to Haight Street. The Haight-Ashbury was locked in a permanent sixties, Grateful Dead, tie-dyed, pot-smoking time warp. I had been a little lost hippie child looking for daddy's love here, and anywhere else I could find it.

Not finding daddy's love on Haight Street, I embarked on a Greyhound bus tour through California and Nevada. South towards Hollywood, then north towards Placerville where a grandmother lived. Next stop, all the way to Carson City, Nevada, where another grandmother lived. I left Carson City abruptly after being propositioned by a short-order cook at the Greyhound bus station. I decided I could do better than him and decided to try my luck once more at Wilbur Hot Springs in Napa Valley.

This time the owner did not insist that I participate in the Health Sanctuary's Gestalt therapy program and work for free (in the seventies, they called this Karma Yoga). He did, however, want to watch me have sex with his wife. Or at the very least, watch them have sex. I wasn't willing to do any of that.

Terrified, I stole a pair of shoes, got caught, and ran again, back to my father's place. His wife didn't want me living there, and so I went to live down the hall with a neighbor who was kind enough to put me up. But after a few weeks the neighbor's generosity faded, and he started dropping not–so–subtle hints that it might be time for me to move on. So I packed up my belongings and had just lugged my suitcase down to the front of the building when I heard someone calling my name.

"Juliet," cried out the male voice. "Do you remember me?" Of course I did. It was this homely photographer I had met while working as a maid at Wilbur Hot Springs. He had taken some nude pictures of me standing near old abandoned mineral baths out in Calistoga, which is near Wilbur Hot Springs. Apparently my modeling abilities had left a lasting impression. Since once again I was on the verge of homelessness, I accepted the photographer's invitation to head out to his home in Santa Cruz.

The photographer made me feel special for a while, a week at least, as he snapped various nude photographs of me. I had sex with him, just like I had sex with anyone I believed could help me out a little. When I wasn't accommodating the photographer I worked on sketches and poetry. My dream of becoming a famous artist comforted me briefly, but then I started bleeding profusely from an abortion I had undergone months before. I was in desperate need of medical attention. To make matters worse, his girlfriend said she needed space. Once again I was not wanted. It seemed like everywhere I turned I was rejected and then abandoned.

Pain and fear choked at my throat as if someone were trying to strangle me. I just wanted someone to love me, but instead all I was getting was a lot of sexual attention that I was not equipped to deal with. I believed that the sexual attention equaled love.

Once, I caught a glimpse of what I thought was love going through Hollywood on yet another Greyhound bus, eating Dorito chips and reading "True Confessions" magazines, wishing that it was me in that story. At the same moment, I looked up into the huge rearview mirror at the front of the bus.

The bus driver smiled at me. His smile warmed me and comforted me.

I was so starved for love and attention that a simple smile from a stranger transformed my visit on that bus. I was home; he was Daddy. I was loved!

I kept looking for that feeling I had in that brief moment while riding that Greyhound bus towards the next city. It was as if I was suspended in space in time, and just for that moment, I was safe, and the pain stopped. But as soon as I got off the bus, the pain and the terror would start up all over again.

Where was I going? Who would take care of me? Why didn't my own father want me? I was beyond frightened—I was terrified down to my very core. From the East Coast to the West Coast, as I bounced back and forth between two sets of parents who did not know how to love me, this experience of fear and isolation followed me wherever I went.

* * *

I believe that when a young person has sex before they are mature enough to really understand what is going on, it can potentially cause psychological damage that lasts a lifetime. Had I believed that I had the right to set sexual boundaries, I would have been spared years of demoralizing degradation.

Incest changed all of that. My stepfather, a learned professor of "Human Sexuality," had positioned himself as an authority on the topic. In the seventies, the new "sexology" advocated prostituting woman. The Sexual Revolution meant women could not say no, that is if they wanted to seem liberated.

The only thing that was liberated was the wallets of the pornographers.

Every day, a child is exploited. Every day, we look the other way. If I did not tell the truth about what happened in my lifetime as a result of my own experiences as an exploited child, it would be as if I too was looking the other way. My stepfather used his stepchildren as sexual surrogates while my suicidal mother looked the other way.

If no one tells the truth, the exploitation will become the norm. Then whoever is exploited will be blamed for what happened to them. They were available for the victimization, showed no resistance, therefore they must have wanted it, and so it's their own fault. *I was blamed for my own victimization by being labeled a bad girl.*

I was defiant, and so I decided that if society viewed me as bad, then I might as well be a good "bad" girl. I shoved my addiction to the sex industry underground, and later it resurfaced as a sex and love addiction.

The only way out of the maze is to tell you the truth. In telling the truth about my sexual experiences I reclaim my womanhood. For too long, first person singular has been told through the eyes of man about woman. I am lifting the veil. This is the journey I took to become whole and reclaim my womanhood.

chapter nine

That night, it was hard for me to sleep. Marie had continued to drink all evening, and it hadn't been a pretty sight. When my sister drank, all hell broke loose. One minute she would be giving you a brilliant lecture on feminist theory, and the next minute she'd be up on the rooftop howling at the moon. Not to mention the fire alarms that seemed to go off for no apparent reason. My sister explained that a poltergeist was responsible. Whatever the explanation, for this and various other odd occurrences that took place while my sister was under the influence, it was painful to watch her drink, especially since I'm a recovering alcoholic.

Besides, I was starting to feel guilty. After all, I was the one who had gone down to the liquor store and bought her another bottle just so that she would give me more information.

I just never could leave well enough alone. I never could stop snooping. My need to find out more information was going to get me in a lot of trouble one day. Actually, it just had, with my own mother. Anyway, once again, I was, in my own way, snooping. I studied the artwork on the wall. Some of it was my own. During my high school days, I had been quite the artiste. Back then, I painted huge, imposing works of art.

A few years later, when I got into college, I put all my paintbrushes in a large sack and gave them away. I had decided I wanted to be an actress. Now, I'm a technical writer in the computer industry. I don't usually tell people about that (it doesn't have a high glamour value).

Sometimes, because of my knowledge of the criminal justice system that I acquired from dealing with my career criminal father, I tell people I am a parole officer for chronic, hardened criminals. Then they forget I ever said I was a technical writer and want to know about the criminal mind.

I can provide information about the criminal mind because I grew up with one, and then, ultimately, became one. While involved in prostitution, I never thought of it as illegal. I am still a thief, however. I steal people's secrets and I hoard them for decades. I don't know why I need to keep going over and over the past. Some might call it self-indulgent. I call it survival. I want to live, and so, to live, I must look into the darkness.

Since I couldn't sleep very well, I started looking through my sister's books. She had a diverse collection. For example, she had books on the Tarot, numerology, and developing psychic abilities. And then there were all the feminist books my sister had acquired, such as Betty Friedan's *The Feminine Mystique*, *Sexual Politics*, by Kate Millett, and *The Female Eunuch* by Germaine Greer.

I wondered if anyone in my age group had even heard of these books, or the authors who wrote them. Each of these books had been a critical dimension in launching the second wave of the women's movement. Unfortunately, if not tragically, it seemed like the women's movement and the fight for equal rights had somehow become cliché and unworthy of either consideration or discussion. And if you dared to have the audacity to say you were a feminist, people just rolled their eyes and yawned. I wondered if there was this big cover-up campaign going on so that everyone forgot the importance of the fight.

While contemplating possible conspiracy theories, I opened up one of my sister's photo albums. I studied the pictures for quite some time. You'll be glad to know I didn't take any of them. But in the past, I have. In fact, I turned the page in the photo album to the exact spot where a picture had formally resided. You could still see the faint outline from the picture, and I bet my sister knew I had taken it. It was a picture taken of me when I was about fourteen, during that horrible week my mother had made a suicide attempt when we were traveling through Europe. We were staying in a small town near Copenhagen, in Denmark. My sister and I used to take turns taking the train into Copenhagen to visit our mother in the psychiatric ward of the hospital. Of course fourteen was a little young to be taking a train, alone, in a foreign country, but in any event, in the picture, I looked sad, and brave, all at once. Once I asked a counselor about why I had stolen this particular picture from my sister's photo album. The counselor said that I was trying to steal back my childhood.

I have also heard that incest survivors are prone to stealing. Still, one is never proud of criminal, or aberrant behavior, no matter what the root underlying cause of it might be. Perhaps one of the reasons that photographs, or family pictures, are so precious to me is that they hold clues. For example, my stepfather used to take pictures of my sister and I constantly. In more than quite a few of these, my sister and I were taking a bath. And then there was the picture taken of me when I was three, dressed in only my underwear. Over the years, in each home that I lived in, I had hung the picture, in its innocent pink frame, on the wall.

But then I started remembering, and the picture didn't seem so innocent anymore. I'll never forget the day I smashed the picture into smithereens. Glass went everywhere. Shards of glass. Fragments of memories. Puzzle pieces I hold up to the light with the hope that upon more careful scrutiny, I will be able to glimpse a hologram of who I once was in the past and thus who I might be now.

When you are a survivor of sexual abuse, bits and pieces of who you are float above and around you. Or, sometimes you hear voices. *Who am I?* The voices shout. *Did this happen? Am I just making this up?*

I put the photo album away and I started thumbing through one of my sister's books (palm reading in five easy lessons). Just then, a yellowing, frayed envelope fell to the floor. Of course, I had to pick it up and look inside. It contained two letters—one from me, and the other from my sister, Marie.

September 1977
Dear Marie:

I am embarrassed at my own apparent lack of knowledge, but what is this war against women you speak of? I knew that women were still fighting for their rights. I knew that we were in what is considered the second wave of the women's movement. I am even sewing a tapestry that says: Equal Rights Amendment 1982.

I am almost eighteen years old. I have felt the weight of sexism lately. I doubt my own power. I wonder who I am. When I was closer to you, and felt the influence of the women's movement, I felt stronger and more able to name whatever it was that I was fighting against.

In my pursuit of total individuality and personal freedom I believed I represented the direction of true liberation for women. I never doubted anything I did or felt.

But lately things are not so in control. Mom and our stepfather think I need to see a psychiatrist, because I'm messing around so much. I start a lot of drawings and paintings and then something gets in the way.

I seem to be vacillating between part time sex symbol and artist. It seems easier to be the girl next door who is desirable and cute and fluffy. I'm scared for my life sometimes. I try to block out this fear by drinking and smoking pot.

I don't know if I can stay in this town. I must write, and paint, or be a famous actress, but I am losing motivation. I am so proud of you for going to College in San Francisco and getting away from Baltimore. If I don't get out of here I'll wind up becoming a hooker on North Charles Street in Baltimore.

I love you and I hope to hear from you soon.

Your sister, Juliet

October 1977

Dear Juliet,

Your letters to me of late have been particularly lacking in details about your life. Where are you, what exactly are you doing? I feel alienated from you—you can't keep giving me intellectual rhetoric about woman as artist, and nothing personal and actual about you and your life, your friends, your loves, difficulties, thoughts.

When you say, "What is this war against women you speak of," it upsets me. Are you serious? Do you mean that you are not aware of the weapon of rape and murder of women, that it has been used for thousands and thousands of years as a tool of oppression? You don't know the scandal and uproar Inez Garcia caused by being the first raped woman to strike out and speak up against rape?

I am sorry for this tone of questioning; I realize it's terrible. But I am shocked that you are so unaware. You should be taking basic feminism with me, and then you would be forced to be more aware. One day I walked out of a lecture in tears from a lurid description of Chinese foot binding, disgusted by the violent pornography they had all over the room.

Enough of this. I just ask you to open your eyes. It is not just "one woman," who has been murdered, as you blithely say, it is millions of *women who have been hurt, or attacked, or demoralized. It has taken me a lot of courage to keep my heart and mind open towards men this semester.*

My first reaction was bitterness and fury and a feeling of utter vulnerability. I went to a women's defense meeting last week, in an attempt to put my anger to use. I am becoming so painfully aware of how little I know about defending myself.

I too feel rootless, lost. Can't stand to live in this limbo, this chaos anymore.

Please write, love, Marie

I clutched the letters to my heart. I had to keep both of them, I just had to. I knew it was terrible for me to once again take mail from family members. First the letter my stepfather had written to my mother, and now these two. But I simply had to have them. Each of the letters provided a reference point, a window into my past.

When I entered the University of Maryland, I had originally planned on a career as an actress, so I selected Visual Performing Arts (theater) as my major. Probably because of my early feminist exposure, I became disillusioned with the world of theater right away. The most common roles for women were either dumb blondes or hookers. What was funny is that this was eventually what I became (a dumb blonde and a hooker).

And here is something even more ironic. Because of all the pot I had smoked in my youth, the unfortunate reality is that I was not really able to reach, artistically speaking, for much more than the proverbial dumb blonde. Anyway, in my freshman year, I was cast as "Peace" in the Greek classic, *Lysistrata*. With my somewhat limited understanding of feminism, I decided that although this part certainly was not that of a dumb-blonde hooker, I was still being typecast. When the cast list was posted on the professor's door, I marked SEXIST! in bold red letters by my name.

Then, fueled by righteous indignation, and a lack of tolerance to the college cafeteria coffee, I proceeded to write angry, brilliant poems about being a teenager in America. Later, I linked these poems together into a play called *MINDRAPE*. It was, essentially, a diatribe against the sexist, misogynistic images of women found in fairy tales, movies and pornography. The main image that had terrified me the most back then was one that ran on the front cover of *Hustler Magazine*, published by the king of smut himself, Larry Flynt. A woman was being fed into a meat grinder!

But the truth is, when I actually had a cast pulled together to perform my feminist play, I was too messed up on drugs to pull it together. I became that which I rebelled against. This had been my self-fulfilling prophecy...

IF I DON'T GET OUT OF HERE I'LL WIND UP BECOMING A HOOKER ON NORTH CHARLES ST. IN BALTIMORE...

Whoregirl

Whoregirl
Whoregirl
So much pain
Walking back to daddy's house
So all alone
Blacked out last night; somewhere
Downtown
San Francisco
On Market Street.

When I got home
I bathed in shame
Someone will find out
Who I really am
Whoregirl.

chapter ten

Leaving San Francisco

The following morning, before anyone was even awake, I made my way, via super shuttle, out of San Francisco. I knew all about super shuttles. I liked super shuttles for the same reason I liked Greyhound buses. They provided quiet anonymity and the comfort that came from knowing I would be moving on to my next destination.

The super shuttle driver turned down Fell Street, which paralleled a strip of the Golden Gate Park called the panhandle. As we passed the corner of Page and Fell Street, I tried to get a look at the old Victorian home I had lived in as a teen with my father. I caught just a fleeting glimpse before the van sped forward.

That old familiar ache pulled at my heart. How many times in my 31 years had I done this very thing—left San Francisco? Left San Francisco only to come back. Every summer of my life I found myself on a plane heading west to San Francisco to once again see my father in California. *California.* Where I always thought that things could be different.

Once I was safely ensconced in the airplane, I pulled out the two letters. I had been seventeen years old, and my sister 23, when the letters were written. We had both been spoon fed the promises and the fury of the second wave of the women's movement. We had no reason to believe that we women couldn't have it all. We said the word feminism with pride. But now feminism is a dirty word.

How did the fiery, passionate feminist, who turned down a role in a college play because I felt I was being type cast as a sex object only a few months later then make a decision to work in the sex industry?

In my search for multiple orgasms and anonymous sex, and still only in my teens and early twenties, it is easy to see how my priorities might have been confused. I turned myself into the very thing I fought against becoming—a dumb blonde hooker. I can understand how my life got off track. But it hardly seemed possible that my sister, once a brilliant scholar who had so passionately announced that there was a war against women, was now in an abusive marriage and unable to stay sober.

Perhaps the women's movement that had inspired my sister and me in the late seventies and early eighties had been eclipsed by the so-called sexual revolution. But now it's 1991, and not the late seventies, and now I'm 31 and my sister is 36. I'm about to be married, for all the wrong reasons, and my sister is a drunk.

* * *

Back in San Diego

I was sprawled out on my living room floor assembling wedding invitations. I was feeling quite intimidated by the whole process. A wedding invitation is made up of several items. In addition to the invitation itself, a tiny slip of tissue paper, the RSVP card and envelope, a blank envelope to contain all that, and then a bigger, fancier envelope on top of that all had to be put together.

Then I worried about how my sister and mother would respond on the RSVP envelope. The wedding was scheduled for December, and I had an overwhelming fear neither one of them was planning on attending.

Several scenes which had taken place over the last few weeks came to mind. My mother burning my stepfather's letter. My sister confirming that I really *had* been sexually abused. Fragments of misplaced memories, like shards of glass piercing my heart, were coming dangerously close to the surface. If I kept thinking about all that, I could well wind up messing up the wedding invitations. So, instead, I started obsessing on Tony again. Tony was the young Latin man I was having a torrid affair with. I put together a few invitations before I came to the realization that obsessing over Tony wasn't going to help me focus any better.

As I listened to the words of the classic Eagles song playing on the radio, I couldn't help but feeling as if I were trapped in my own "Hotel California." I turned the dial of the radio and, as the words of the Eagles song echoed through my head, I tried to let go of my latest obsession. But I couldn't do it. I simply couldn't stop thinking about him. Tony. Gorgeous Tony, with the dark, curly hair, and sexy Caribbean accent, and those sweet lips. He reminded me of a piece of chocolate wrapped inside of a shiny, cellophane wrapper.

I simply had to find out what was underneath the wrapping. Then as soon as I did, I'd stare at the smooth, chocolate surface. And then, I had no choice; powerless, I took that first bite. For a moment, the mouth watering, sugary chocolate gave me great pleasure. But then, inevitably, a feeling of emptiness followed. Surely I just needed more chocolate—wasn't that it?

In the "Big Book" of *Alcoholics Anonymous,* in a chapter entitled "The Doctor's Opinion," the doctor describes a "phenomenon of craving," whereupon taking the first drink sets in motion a physical allergic reaction coupled with an insatiable craving in the mind.

As a love addict, I believe my first kiss, as it were, is comparable to engaging in that first drink. I craved that first kiss like an alcoholic craved the first tall, frosty, long necked bottle of Budweiser beer. The first kiss made me high. It was wrong, I would tell myself, to be caught up in a whirlwind affair, especially only *months* before one's wedding. I knew that—and yet even though I was trying to stop, it seemed I was powerless over my actions.

For example, just a couple of weeks ago, desperate for Tony's attention, I agreed to have sex with him and one of his friends, while another one of his crew looked on. Then once we were "finished," Tony waved a vile of cocaine in front of me, despite his knowledge that I was clean and sober.

In one evening, I had jeopardized both my sobriety from drugs and alcohol and my wedding engagement. The next morning I felt hung over. I felt humiliated…dirty. But that didn't stop me. The following night I was back at "Kix." One of Tony's homeboys came up to me and informed me that I "Sure give lousy head."

I was crushed. Demoralized. My life had been reduced to a veritable stranger's opinion of how well I gave a blowjob. What had happened to me? Why was I acting out like this? If only I knew then what I know now. That my acting out was a direct result of the sexual abuse I'd suffered, through my childhood, adolescence, and into an adulthood scarred by my involvement in the sex industry.

That incident got my attention, and shortly after that night, I had composed a passionate, melodramatic letter explaining to Tony that our affair was over, and I wouldn't be able to see him again. *Like he even cared.* And then, in order to cope with the painful withdrawals that immediately set in, I began to scheme about how to start the next affair. Of course, it never occurred to me that this would only exacerbate my problems.

While in the grip of the obsession, *I truly believed* that I had to have as many affairs as I could right up to the wedding day. I felt I owed it to myself. After all, I reasoned, once I was married, I wouldn't have affairs anymore.

And so I proceeded to peruse my little "black book" in order to secure my next hostage. At one point, I even contacted one of my previous employers, hoping to connect with an old boyfriend who used to work there. I struck out in locating him, but that did nothing to deter me from my relentless quest for trapping the next lover, the next *fix* in order to ease my mounting sense of desperation.

I was a love vampire who constantly needed new blood. One night, after returning home from the local nightclub, I played back my messages. There were several from my fiancé, who was out of town on business. He was understandably upset that I wasn't home. And although I was well aware there might be dire consequences as a result of my uncontrollable acting out, I absolutely *could not stop.*

I simply *had* to look for the next fix, and capture the next man. Man A was no longer in the picture, which meant I would have to find Man B. Looking back, I realize that I stored men in the closet like an alcoholic might stash secret bottles in their closet. I always kept a multitude of men who I would file away as "rain checks."

At this point, I had lost all power of choice. I simply *had* to find the next lover. I lived completely for the thrill of romance, the total thrill of the forbidden. The pattern was in my veins. After all, hadn't my father been chasing other women while I was still in my mother's womb? Hadn't he run off with our sixteen year old babysitter? Surely betrayal must somehow be etched into my DNA.

One night, Patrick wanted to go out dancing.

"Let's go to Kix," he insisted. "After all, you seem to love that place so much."

"Kix," I stammered, my heart racing. "You don't want to go to there…no one goes there anymore. That place has really gone downhill."

"Oh is that right," he snapped at me. "Well then why the hell are you so fascinated with it?"

"I just like to dance, that's all."

"Yeah, right," he said. "Get ready, because we're going."

Deep down, what happened is what every addict dreads the most. The inevitable colliding of my secret, hidden world, with my other world, the real world. My heart pounding, we walked into the nightclub. Ironically enough, I wore white.

THERE SHE IS—IT'S THAT ENGAGED WOMAN WHO IS HAVING AFFAIRS…I knew that's what everyone was thinking. I WAS EVIL. A BAD GIRL. A SEXUAL GIRL.

We danced a couple of dances. I was terrified. Any minute someone would come up to me and then Patrick would know the truth. That I was an unfaithful woman. Or any minute someone would walk in and see me with my fiancé and realize that I wasn't single like I pretended to be.

"I'm sorry Patrick," I said. "I just don't feel like dancing."

"I thought you loved dancing," Patrick said, practically hissing at me.

"I do," I said, my sense of horror increasing as I saw Tony walk by with several members of his all-boy gang. "I'm just feeling a little dizzy; can we sit down a minute?"

After we sat down, I was having a hard time focusing on anything but Tony and his entourage. I had this terrible feeling that they were talking about the episode the other night, and how I, as his friend claimed, "Didn't give very good head."

I felt myself fragmenting, splitting off, as I remembered the humiliating event.

"Why are you staring at those guys like that?" Patrick said, bringing me back to reality.

"Was I staring?" I said, genuinely startled. "I didn't mean to, I guess I'm not feeling very well."

"You're staring at them because you're a tramp," Patrick said, becoming red in the face. He stood up from the table and grabbed me by the arm. "We're leaving."

When we were driving home, I knew it was true. I was a BAD GIRL. A TRAMP. After all, hadn't my stepfather told me that my entire life? I closed my eyes, and there he was…

"You're a whore," my stepfather used to say. "Just a filthy whore. That's all you'll ever amount to. It's your fault I did the things I did to you. You asked for it…all you tramps do."

For so many years, my sister and I believed my stepfather's lies. We told ourselves we must have deserved the abuse. Deserved his probing fingers. We swallowed his guilt, unaware that this guilt was poisonous. I can still hear his voice…

Your fault. It's your fault I did the things I did to you. You asked for it…

As a young girl, I made a decision. If everyone told me I was a bad girl, I would be the best bad girl there was. Even in junior high and high school, I had a reputation. I was a slut. In every school there was at least one girl everyone knew was a slut. I was that girl. If you were promiscuous, you were exiled by other girls, used for boy's sexual pleasures, and then cast aside. I didn't know any other way.

That night, after we got back from the nightclub, Patrick and I made love. Only it really wasn't making love, and it never was. It was sex. And if we weren't engaged it would almost seem like rape. But I knew down to my core that I deserved this. I was not there as he moved in and out of me. I really did not want to be sexual with him, but I knew I had no choice.

This is what was expected of me. I felt myself splitting off. There, suspended safely above our sexual exchange I began to crawl into my imaginary glass cage. It was very dark in our room, but in my glass cage, it was very light, almost pleasant.

I felt oblivion for a few pleasurable minutes, but then, for the second time that day, I heard it. My stepfather's voice.

You're nothing but a whore.
She's a bad girl! She'll runaway before she is sixteen.
You'll never be anything but a tramp.

After Patrick was finished having sex with me, I stared up at the ceiling and tried to forget about the voice I had heard. Would I ever stop hearing his voice? I tried to ignore my sense of panic and I wondered what was wrong with me. I wondered if this is what it would be like to be married to Patrick. My body would not be my own. Instead, it would become an instrument leased out in exchange for financial security. I would be a whore wearing a fancy wedding ring.

I told myself that it was okay that my sexual needs were not taken into consideration in tonight's session with Patrick. As the perfect bride-to-be, I was to sacrifice my pleasure so that my future husband would be happy.

In the Victorian Age, women who enjoyed sex were considered evil, or animalistic. Then, if a woman did not enjoy sex, and was sickly, pale, and passive, she was considered to be ultra-feminine. Next, she was placed on a pedestal, where she froze to death.

But that was then, and now, the tigress danced within. I tossed and turned, wide awake. My own orgasm, or lack thereof, had always been of paramount importance to me. While I was in my teens, I had never had an orgasm, and in the seventies, that was like saying you couldn't breathe. I was absolutely terrified of my orgasmless state.

After all, I had grown up reading *True Confessions* magazine, and books like *The Story of O*. In *The Story of O*, the woman's main purpose was to be a sexual slave, a receptacle for her male master's fantasies. In all of these stories, women convulsed with multiple orgasms as soon as the male entered them in the customary missionary position.

Years later, when I decided to become a writer, I thought perhaps it would be easier to get published if I wrote Romance Novels. Silhouette Intimate Moments, or Harlequin True Romance novels in hand, I hunkered down to read, sure that the formula would be easy to duplicate. The part that was easiest to duplicate was the romance genre's treatment of the sexual experience. Each heroine climaxed the instant the male penis thrust into them.

Well, I've never climaxed that way, I thought. *I needed direct clitoral stimulation.* And I needed it for more than five minutes. The clitoris is my friend. Anyway, as my fiancé slept, I twisted and turned, and, extremely sexually dissatisfied, I began to plot a way to get Tony back. One of my other personas took over, and I wasn't even in the room.

* * *

One day, I stumbled into a recovery group that began my journey of sexual healing. I had actually been looking for an AA meeting when I happened to walk by a room with a sign posted on the door. The sign said, "Sex and Love Addicts Anonymous Meeting In Session." I had walked past that room before. *Now those people really must have a problem,* I always thought.

But today, perhaps out of my own desperation, I had a more receptive, open mind. Today, I did not walk past the meeting room. Instead, I took a deep breath and went in.

"This is the San Diego Bottom Line Getting Current Meeting, I'm Jason, and I'm a sex and love addict; oh, I'm also the secretary of your meeting," he said, grinning.

"Hi Jason," the group said, as I slid into a seat, hoping nobody noticed me.

Jason smiled in my direction, and continued talking. "Your bottom line behavior is any sexual or emotional act, which once engaged in, leads to a loss of control. Staying away from this behavior defines sobriety. One day at a time, we don't act out. We don't practice behaviors which lead to a loss of control."

The secretary then introduced the leader, who started the meeting. "Hi, I'm Denise," she said, tossing a wild mane of blonde hair. "I'm a sex and love addict."

"Hi, Denise," everyone said.

"I was in the sex industry," Denise said frankly. "I was a prostitute. I'm no longer in the sex industry but I'm having affairs and I think my marriage is just about over."

I couldn't *believe* her honesty. I couldn't believe that she had openly admitted to being both a prostitute and having affairs. I continued to stare at this woman. How could she do that? How could she possibly admit to these behaviors?

Despite her radical admission, the meeting proceeded. Other people in the room introduced themselves and spoke about their addiction. These are a few of the comments I heard that day.

"I'm married—that is, I *was* married. My husband caught me in bed with another man. Now I'm heading for divorce court."

"I masturbate constantly, sometimes for hours at a time until it becomes painful."

"I have one night stands almost every night."

"I am addicted to pornography."

"I'm a stripper and I always choose abusive relationships."

Encouraged by the group's honesty, I decided to share as well. "I'm engaged, and yet I can't stop having affairs. I keep trying to, but there is always one more reason why I have to start something up again." Everyone nodded. I felt understood and accepted. And so I continued. "My relationship with my fiancé gets worse and worse because I'm totally preoccupied with the other guy. But the other guy keeps standing me up. Every time he does it I tell myself I won't see him again, but then I think, I'll give it one more chance. Then he promised me a gold bracelet and so now I'm obsessed with getting it. He says if he can watch me with another woman he'll give me the gold bracelet.

"That part of my behavior worries me because it—" *It reminds me of the same behavior I had when I was a prostitute,* I thought, but the words froze in my throat. The people in the meeting were staring at me, hanging on my every word, or so it seemed to me. "Well, I just know it isn't right, since I'm not really bisexual, at least now that I'm sober from drugs and alcohol." I felt myself turning a deep shade of red. Shame surged through me. Why had I just revealed the intimate details of my secret, hidden world to these people?

After the meeting had concluded, I was one of the first people out the door. I heard one of the meeting members calling my name. I glanced behind me; it was that woman Denise who had openly discussed her former career in the sex industry.

"Juliet!" she shouted excitedly. "Juliet! There's something I wanted to talk to you about."

I pretended I didn't hear her and fled to my car. *Why had I run away from that woman?* I wondered. While driving home, I started thinking about some of the things I had heard during the meeting.

Then, I thought about this boyfriend I had cut loose right before I got sober. His name was Armando, and he claimed to be a Portuguese Mafia drug dealer. Eventually I found out what a womanizer he was. He had a girlfriend named Meth, as in Crystal Meth. He pushed me to be sexual with her, and other women.

As I had mentioned to the Sex and Love Addicts Anonymous group, I did not consider myself to be bisexual by nature. A child of the "sexual revolution," of course I experimented with it, but unless drugs or money were part of the scenario, it wasn't my normal tendency. Usually my choice to be "bisexual" was based on wanting to fulfill a male's fantasy, and he had either a) lot's of cocaine, or b) lot's of money, or c) a combination of both (a) and (b).

After I got sober, all bisexual activity ceased. Armando called for months trying to set up sexual fantasies that involved me and other girls. Once, I accidentally picked up one of his calls and he started going on and on about this seventeen year old who knew how to do things with ice that I really should see. I explained to him that I was sober now and I was trying to live a different kind of life. I knew that I couldn't carry on that way anymore if I wanted to stay sober. *Why wasn't I able to make the same connections now?* I wondered, as I took the exit marked Mission Valley.

The weekly routine in our home went about like this. Patrick worked in Ventura all week, and at night, he stayed at a Motel 6. He would come home during the weekends. We were planning to maintain this arrangement until after the wedding, at which point we would both move to Ventura. Anyway, in what was a typical example of our schedule, one morning Patrick packed up his things to drive out to Ventura. Every night, he would try to call me from his hotel room, and more often than not, I wasn't home.

I wasn't home because I was out on the prowl. Because no matter how I dressed it up, I was addicted to sex and love. I got a high from being in love. I got a euphoric rush when I knew a man wanted me. And the kind I liked the best were the dangerous ones. Bad boys. Men with tattoos and checkered pasts and a mean look in their eyes. Men who looked the other way. Men, who, to use the parlance of the times, were emotionally unavailable. Men like Tony.

I am engaged, and yet I spend most of my time obsessing on Tony. *Why isn't he ever where he says he will be? Why does he constantly stand me up? Why do I allow him to? When will we have sex again?* I am hooked into a cycle of lust, abandonment and rejection that I believe I am powerless to change. And the pain that I was experiencing as a result of this acting out was absolutely excruciating.

And so instead of the relationship with my husband-to-be, I was thinking of getting that gold bracelet from Tony. I never considered that what I was contemplating doing in return for that bracelet might be classified as turning a trick. Instead, I was only thinking of the heady sense of power the bracelet would give me.

I was trained by my stepfather at a very young age that material items equaled love. Like many perpetrators, my stepfather used material items to both buy our silence and ensure compliance. Once, upon returning from a trip he had taken to Africa with my mother, my stepfather brought us back little gold masks on a gold chain. Then, from another trip, to Hawaii, he brought back gold leaves, also on gold chains, which were popular in the seventies. Or stereos for Christmas. Fine gifts. Gifts that got our attention.

She's nothing but a whore.
She'll runaway when she's sixteen.

After being gone all week as usual, Patrick and I were taking a Saturday morning walk on the paths surrounding the river tributaries that ran through Mission Valley in San Diego.

"I'm not sure I have sexual feelings anymore," I admitted.

"What the hell are you talking about?" he snarled.

"I just don't feel that sexual towards you when you're always so angry at me."

"Maybe if you stopped running around," he shot back at me.

"I just like to go out dancing—"

"Save it," he said. "You'll never change."

And so it went. Our fights were often so vicious that people walking by stared at us to make sure I was okay. Patrick would basically attack everything about me—my beliefs, my political orientation, my religious understanding—all of these were fair game for his scrutiny and put-downs. During the assaults, I would shut down. After all, I had grown up with verbal and emotional terrorism, so perhaps it seemed familiar to me. Surely it would get better once we were married. All I had to do was deny my sexual past and become a goodgirl. Then he would not be so cruel.

It's not that bad. He doesn't really mean it, I told myself. *Besides,* I tried to convince myself, *I don't care. I just don't care.* But deep down, I did care. And so did the little girl within me. She was crying out for recognition. But I had learned to shut her out. If I could have listened to her, maybe I would have heard her pain, and her concern that I was rushing into a marriage that was going to fit me about as well as my last one did, in other words, not at all.

I was using affairs to get a fix, to gloss over my intolerable reality. Vaguely, just vaguely, I sensed that I was locked into a pattern. But I had no idea of the desperate seriousness of my condition. I had created, once again, a double world. I had one life on the outside as a young, college educated about to be married woman. On the surface I was going along with all the wishes of my future husband. But I had a hidden world, another life that I lived behind his back. I had hidden agendas. Secret plans. Hidden trysts to carry out. Old hurts to run from.

Deep down, although I was out of the sex industry, I still felt like a whore spiritually. How could I have known, how could I have possibly understood that I was suffering from very severe post-traumatic stress disorder no different from that of a Vietnam vet?

chapter eleven

1978
Baltimore

It's not like you wake up one morning and think, "Oh, I'd like to be in the sex industry." It was the late seventies. I was living downtown, and I desperately needed money for college and for rent. I was terrified. It was winter...

One day, a girl I had gone to high school with pulled up in front of my apartment building on North Charles St. driving a red Mercedes Benz. "Ever been in one of these?" Penelope said.

I shook my head. As a matter of fact, my usual mode of transportation was the bus. Riding public transportation usually turned out to be a unique cultural experience for me, since I was generally the only white person present.

"Wanna go for a ride?" asked Penelope.

I didn't have anything else to do, except for the usual, like find a job, and probably a different place to live. Normally, I was either hung over or under the influence when I went calling on possible job locations, and therefore did not make a lasting impression. I had been using drugs and drinking since I was thirteen. During all of my teen years there was always some combination of drugs and alcohol in my system.

My self-destructive choices and my untreated drug and alcohol addiction were very much related. And so, because I knew Penelope usually had some decent drugs in her possession, I said "Why not?" and climbed in.

It was my first time in a Mercedes Benz, and I felt a little out of place.

"I'm worth more than you," she said, navigating through traffic.

"What are you talking about?" I asked.

"I'm living with Baltimore's most important hair stylist and I'm driving his car."

I didn't say a word. What could I say—on the surface she appeared to be right. I was flat broke, and it showed. While most of my clothes came from thrift stores, all of Penelope's clothes looked brand new. I was not unfamiliar with hunger, in fact, my stomach was growling, and I was wondering if she would be buying us lunch since she was doing so well.

I flashed on the last time I had seen Penelope—about a year ago—in San Francisco. I was sixteen. Once again, my father couldn't be bothered with me. A male neighbor who lived down the hall had been kind enough to put me up for a while. Penelope showed up with this black guy; I had no idea that he was her pimp.

Even back then, I had the vague awareness that Penelope was going down the wrong track. But now she was "worth" more than me.

"My boyfriend has connections," she bragged.

"Like who?" I said, as we drove around downtown Baltimore in the red Mercedes.

"He knows this lady named Angela. She's a madam. Have you ever heard of a madam?"

"I think so," I said. "It's a woman who gets prostitutes for men."

"Sort of, but a real madam is much more sophisticated than that."

"How?" I asked.

"I'm talking about a real high class madam who gets call girls for rich guys. Call girls aren't prostitutes. They're higher class than that."

"Oh, I get it," I said. And now I felt even more out of place. Even the smell of the car was completely foreign to me. I must seem so naïve to my friend.

"Well, my boyfriend introduced me to Angela. And she'd like to meet you."

I felt a tiny thrill. "Me, she wants to meet me?"

My friend nodded, regal as she effortlessly steered the large luxury car through downtown Baltimore.

I started working for the madam that week. It was a simple matter of meeting her in a coffee shop. She looked me over, asked me for my measurements, and said, "When can you start?"

* * *

Winter, 1980
Baltimore

The temperatures had reached record lows that winter in Baltimore. By noon it was still no warmer than a frigid eleven degrees. I sat in the front room of Angela's apartment. Bored, I lifted the gold brocade drapes and looked out.

"What the hell are you doing?" demanded Angela, grabbing my wrist. She held on tightly, the tops of her nails digging into my wrists.

"Let me go," I cried out.

"Well then let go of that curtain," she snarled.

I dropped the curtain and Angela released my hand. My skin burned where her nails had dug into my wrists and my eyes filled with salty tears.

Angela just stood there, glaring at me. "There's no reason for you to cry," she finally said, her voice heavy with contempt.

"You hurt me."

"Let me see your wrist." She glared at my wrist and then flung it away. "You'll live."

I had been working for the madam for almost three years now. I was almost 21. "You know," Angela said, as she whisked through the apartment, straightening ashtrays, "All it takes is being seen once by the wrong person, and we're out of business. You don't want that to happen do you?"

She methodically placed her souvenir New Jersey pillow so that it looked neat yet casual next to her Niagara Falls souvenir pillow.

"No, Angela," I said, sitting rigidly in my chair, "I don't."

"You've got a one o'clock and a two o'clock appointment," Angela told me.

"Okay."

"Did you get that garter set I told you about?"

"No, I'm sorry, I didn't."

She sat down in a gold easy chair across from me and hastily dabbed out her elongated menthol cigarette.

I took in the visage of the woman before me. Thin lips pulled downward in an angry crescent moon shape. Flaming red hair, which she had washed and set every week in an exclusive salon, framed a too pale face. There were black and blue marks around her eyes from recent plastic surgery.

"That's the second time this week I've reminded you about the garter set."

Jesus Christ, I'm thinking. *There's something wrong with this picture.*

I'm the sweet young wrinkle-free thing she gets to auction off to the highest bidder so she can get plastic surgery and she's all obsessed with the garter set. Like most of the guys really care what I have on.

She shook her head and filed a long, dagger shaped nail painted fire engine red. "And please, Juliet, remember to put out a fresh hand towel in the bathroom after every client leaves. You forgot to put them out after your first appointment this morning."

"Yeah, sure," I mumbled. Like she couldn't put the towels out herself. I'm the one who does the dirty work and she gets half and then she wants me to put a towel out. "I guess I keep forgetting."

"It's the dope you smoke," Angela said.

"It's your dope, Angela," I replied angrily.

"Don't you dare contradict me," she shouted, the palm of her hand moving towards me.

I pulled away, stammering. "I wasn't contradicting you, I just—"

"I can't have any trouble here. And let me tell you something, Miss Hotpants, if you don't start taking your job a little more seriously, I'll let you go. This is a business, like working in a bank or an office, and I like things done a certain way. Do you understand?"

I just looked at her. She was crazy. There was no doubt about it. What other explanation could there be for her mistreatment of me? She didn't treat the other girls like that. How did she think she paid for her plastic surgery? She paid for it with the money I grossed for her during just one week. I knew for a fact I was pulling in more money than any girl ever did. Angela, who always prided herself on being a top-notch businesswoman, apparently didn't know the first thing about the bottom line.

"I said, do you understand?"

"Yeah, I mean, yes ma'am, I understand."

"Make sure you do, because believe me, you can be easily replaced."

Oh, well, I thought, as I flipped through the pages of

Cosmopolitan for the third time that morning. *At least I wasn't a common street hooker.* I was protected; I was a high-class call girl, after all. I read an article on greater orgasmic power, and wondered why I had never in my life experienced anything like that. Actually, even though I was now a call girl, I was terrified of sex. I just had to take a lot of drugs so that I didn't care.

Anyway, I picked up a paperback copy of *The Happy Hooker*, by Xaviera Hollender that Angela proudly displayed on her coffee table. You could tell she'd really studied the book carefully. Some of the pages from the book were dog-eared and she had even highlighted certain passages.

Ms. Hollender, who also had a column in *Penthouse* magazine, made promiscuity and prostitution seem highly desirable. First of all, Xaviera never felt guilty about charging for sex. Not only that, she had multiple orgasms—with every trick! I had never even had an orgasm yet. Or at least I wasn't sure if I had. I was pretty sure that I hadn't.

And so, as I sat there, in Angela's tacky little living room, reading about Xaviera's multiple orgasms, I made a decision. *I wanted to be just like Xaviera Hollender.* I put the book down, thinking. It had been hard to ask for money at first. But men always drifted to me like honeybees, so I started charging a price for my honey. Wasn't that the American way? Xaviera didn't feel badly about it so why should I?

The Happy Hooker glorified all aspects of prostitution. Compelled, I picked up the book once more. Xaviera's sexual powers seemed unlimited. Could anyone really have that many orgasms and get paid for it too?

"Charlotte, you better clean up for your appointment," Angela said.

Charlotte was my working name. We ladies of leisure (another misnomer) never used our real names. "Who is it?" I asked.

"It's our staff gynecologist, Dr. George."

As far as I could tell, all the tricks thought they were gynecologists. Angela always told all the clients that Dr. George regularly examined us once a month for sexually transmitted diseases, but that was just a big fat lie. Dr. George had never examined me, at least not for diseases.

I didn't say anything. Instead, I went into the bathroom and douched with FreshFlowers. Before and after every trick, I douched. It was the least I could do.

Then, I thought about the time Dr. George had me meet him in what is known as a trick pad. It's a place that john's lease or rent for their "dates" with girls like me. Anyway, Dr. George was kind enough to come fully equipped with a syringe filled with Valium. Since I was always a little like Alice in Wonderland and felt it was my duty to try all new drugs, I said sure, beam me up. Thank God, it was the first and last time I used a needle. And what if it hadn't really been Valium? What if it had been heroin?

Anyway, after I was well sedated, the good doctor proceeded to test drive his pop-up dick. I'm not kidding. He had a popup dick. Apparently, he had used the money he had earned by exploring other women's anatomy to buy himself a penile implant. Even with the implant, which he activated with a small button, it was hard not to notice that his penis, was, well, rather abbreviated. *When you are a prostitute there are always so many things that you have to pretend you don't notice. Your whole life, for instance.*

But that was then, and right now, I had a job to do, so I went into Angela's room. It was crowded with baroque furniture, nude cupid sculptures, more souvenir pillows and shelves filled with sharp glass objects. There was no apparent order; chaos reigned amidst this wreckage of gaudy trinkets, bangles and bracelets.

I selected a black garter belt and stockings from out of the bottom drawer of an overstuffed dresser. I stood and watched myself dress in front of an oval, standing mirror. I'm not sure—maybe there was a distortion in the mirror. Because even though I was on the petite side, I believed right then that I looked as fat as a stuck pig. And then I had a really difficult time attaching the stockings to the garter belt. Maybe I just wasn't doing it right, but I just couldn't get the loop over the little clasp.

As I stood there in front of the mirror, fumbling with the garters, I had this whirling, spinning sensation, like I was falling. I felt like I was standing outside of myself, watching a movie. *This isn't real. You're just playing a role,* I told myself, as I finally managed to attach the garter to the stocking.

I moved about the room, trying to shake myself from whatever had just happened. It was probably just the drugs, I thought. I simply hadn't mixed the right combination. In the next room, I listened to Angela as she conducted heavy-duty public relations over the phone.

"Oh, it's you," she gushed, her voice grainy and saccharine sweet. "I've got my college co-ed here today. I swear she could be Miss Maryland. She's a 34-B. Yes, she is on the thin side, just the way you like. Blonde and petite, and just as sweet as she is pretty."

I have to tell you, it's really strange to listen to someone advertising a product, when that product is you. But I knew, as I floated around the room, that nothing mattered. I wasn't even really here; the downer I had begged Angela to give me was starting to kick in.

"Four o'clock? Sure. We'll see you then."

I quickly calculated what another customer would be worth. I had already had five other dates today. That's what you called them. Dates. Probably so you wouldn't have to feel so bad about what they really were—tricks. Anyway, I earned fifty dollars per date. Angela made the same amount.

Here she was, demanding a fifty percent cut and then going on and on about putting a fresh hand towel in the bathroom for each customer. Like it would really kill her to go ahead and do it herself. And sometimes she even tried to cheat me out of my money. I wouldn't notice until the next day, when I sobered up a little.

And by then it was too late to accuse her of anything; she would just laugh in my face. One thing was for sure, I knew that if I wanted to stay on top of her game, I would have to stay straight—no drugs or alcohol. But I knew that wasn't possible. That would make this whole deal way too real.

Angela opened the door and peered imperiously at me. "Are you almost ready?"

"Yes. Should I stay in here?"

She nodded. "As soon as he finishes his drink I'll bring him in."

I took out my vial of coke. I opened the tiny bottle and scooped out some of the white powder with a tiny spoon. The drug surged through my brain, lighting a fire in my womb, igniting a false feeling of horniness.

Suddenly I was Xaviera Hollender, and I just couldn't wait to have sex. Once again, I looked at my reflection in the mirror. Only this time, I didn't look fat. I looked pretty good, if I did say so myself. I licked a finger and rubbed it along one of the breasts that swelled out of the black push-up bra. Then I traced a fingernail just underneath the edge of my stocking.

I was ready now.

I smiled seductively at the next client, but then something weird happened. I looked at this guy and I saw the face of my stepfather. All of a sudden I wasn't feeling very well, and I rushed into the bathroom. I could hear Angela trying to make excuses for me, and I knew the guy was pissed. I really wasn't sure how I would get through this. I splashed water on my face, and then did another line. So far, I wasn't having a very good day.

When I went back into the bedroom, the client was waiting, undressed, on the bed. "Play with yourself little girl," he instructed.

And so I did. I felt pretty embarrassed about it, but it's not like I had any choice about the matter. I had a job to do like anyone else. After awhile, I stopped, and the client nodded at me, which I knew was my cue to give him head. I really wasn't that good at giving head, if you want to know the truth. I wasn't that good at it because, in general, it made me want to gag. But if I didn't give him head I wouldn't get paid. It didn't take a rocket scientist to figure that out.

And so I began working on him, all the while moaning like I was having the time of my life.

The men who came into the madam's bedroom had no faces. They had sex with me and then when they were finished they sat up and smoked or told stories. Each man always had his own story, you know, the reason he was here. It was usually the same thing—their wives or girlfriends did not excite them anymore.

And then they always wanted to know what a nice girl like me was doing here. As if it mattered. And so I told them the same story. That I wanted to be an artist and I was making my way through college. Each man always wanted my phone number. I had to tell them that I wasn't allowed to give out my phone number and please not to take it personally. If I gave them my number, the madam could fire me for trying to steal her clientele. It's your loss they would indignantly reply, and I would assure them that yes, it truly was my loss.

All day long they licked me, prodded me, fucked me, told me I was special, that I wasn't like the other girls—when really I was just a whore. Some of them even liked to tell me that they loved me, especially when they started to come. I always wondered why they even bothered with all that. They could never love a girl like me.

Perhaps they tried to make it more than it was out of their own guilt over seeing a prostitute. If they could convince themselves, even for a moment, that they cared about me, they could postpone their own sense of shame. But most of them just did their business and rolled off of me, used their hand towels, put back on their suit and ties, and walked away. No emotional attachments. That was part of the deal. I understood that better than when they tried to get romantic on me.

I could be any girl; they do not care as long as I have a vagina.

I lay underneath them and I quietly hate myself for allowing so many men to have sex with me. And I hate them for wanting to. It hurts. I spend so much time convincing myself that this life is okay, when I know damn well it's killing me.

chapter twelve

1981
Baltimore

I wanted out. For over three years, I had been working for the madam. Having managed to work my way through college by turning tricks, I felt that finally the time had come to leave behind the double life I'd led for so long: college co-ed by day, prostitute—no, excuse me, "call-girl" by night.

I sat watching Princess Diana and Prince Charles' wedding on the madam's small TV. As I watched, I knew without question that I wanted to be like Princess Diana. Actually, what I really wanted was to have a Prince Charles to rescue me from my sordid existence.

Even though I was working as a prostitute, I was still living with my mother. She had finally left a marriage of 17 years to my abusive stepfather, and since then we had spent nearly a year living in a small apartment outside of Baltimore. But then, after my mother decided to marry one of our neighbors, a man who lived downstairs, once again, I had to make new living arrangements.

At the time, my addiction to the sex industry was at its height. I was on a "sugar-daddy hunt." Regular tricks weren't good enough for me. No. I wanted men to "keep me," or, in other words, pay my rent. For example, I remember trying, rather unsuccessfully I might add, to hustle a senior-citizen trick who owned topless bars in Baltimore. "Don't you like the way I cut my hair?" I asked. And, "I'm wearing the perfume you said you liked," I let him know.

"I already have a mistress," he finally explained.

"How old is she?" I asked the perspective sugar daddy. I couldn't understand why he didn't want to buy me, make me his possession. After all, I was one heck of a deal. White. Blonde. Petite. A perfect sexual wind-up doll—and at such a bargain price.

"If you must know, she's 27."

"Well I'm only 21," I pleadingly replied, in a further attempt to negotiate.

The "john" wasn't impressed, which, at that time, baffled me. He did, however, offer to help me qualify for the rental agreement on my mother's apartment. I had decided to try and stay there, even after my mother moved out. All he had to do was tell the rental office that I worked for him, which at some obscure level was actually the truth. You see, I had been earning plenty of income, but my kind of income didn't show up on a TRW report, if you know what I mean.

In the end, the man who owned the topless bars (and was old enough to be my grandfather) didn't help me qualify for an apartment like he said he would. Why was it so hard to find a sugar daddy? I wondered. All the prospective sugar daddy had to do was pretend to be my father, pay my rent, and maybe stick some braces on my teeth. I had this overbite that my parents had never bothered to correct, and I was always trying to convince tricks to buy me braces. So far, none had, but that didn't stop me from trying.

And so, one day, I sat on my suitcase in my mother's empty apartment. I was trying to push my overbite in with my left thumb. I figured if I just did this a few minutes a day, say for the next twenty years, maybe my two bucked teeth would move in and become less noticeable. But beyond getting my teeth fixed, I needed a plan, and I needed one fast. I had to figure out where I was going to live, and how I was going to survive.

I was scared. I knew what poverty felt like. I had walked down city streets with nothing but my portable typewriter, my beat-up suitcase that had formally belonged to my father, and my dreams.

While this might have sounded brave and poetic, I didn't want to live that way ever again. And so, rather than face homelessness again, I decided to accept my first fiancé's marriage proposal. After all, Craig had been pestering me for over a year to marry him. Up until now, I just wasn't sure that I loved him enough to marry him. All of a sudden, when I thought of warm sunny California, where Craig now lived, I started to feel more amorous by the minute. Besides, all I had to do was make a phone call, and within days, an airline ticket would show up in the mail. At that time, it seemed as if it were the easiest decision I had ever made.

chapter thirteen

*The Eighties
California!*

My new life in California started out as a delightful, sun-splashed paradise in comparison to dreary, sleazy Baltimore. Our apartment complex, which had been constructed in a perfect circle, was comparable to living in a perfectly contained oasis. Palm trees flowing in the sultry warm breeze. Bright orange hibiscus flowers. A pool, jacuzzi, and tennis courts right inside that perfect circle. Even the air smelled sweet, fragrant from the variety of tropical flowers and shrubs which, in California, were in bloom year round.

All I needed to do was loll by the pool, make sure my tan lines were in place, and figure out whether or not I should go to Jazzercise or aerobics. I was in love with San Diego, and even more in love with California living.

On the other hand, I wasn't so sure about married life.

The day we got married, the Major, husband number one's

father, gave me away. He was nicknamed this due to the fact that he had been a major in the marines. At the time, I felt it was kind of the Major to give me away, since I secretly believed I was "damaged goods." In fact he was so kind, he allowed us to move into his palatial home overlooking eastern San Diego.

I had arrived! I was an American Princess Diana!! I left behind a life of sleazy filthy Baltimore alleys, overweight, aging sugar daddies who wouldn't even agree to be my sugar daddies, and my sordid, secret life as a sex worker.

When I hit the working world in the early eighties, I guess you could say I had something to prove. My new father-in-law suggested I take up technical writing in the computer industry. I didn't know what else to do, so I decided to try it. My first job in the computer industry was as a proofreader. Although it was a big adjustment for me to enter the corporate world, I was grateful to be in a professional work environment that was legal, where the only viruses were in the computers and not from diseases.

I entered the computer industry as soon as I got out of college, which was in 82. I was 22 years old. Other than the Feminist Theory and Women's Studies classes I had taken in school, I really hadn't retained very much. After all, I had been either stoned or drunk ever since I was 13 years old. The only reason I really graduated from college was because it was a very "liberal" liberal arts college. The theater professors gave me A's for my plays, and eventually my journalism professor thought I turned out some good material. Even my composition teacher in my college years took me aside and told me I had some writing talent.

I wasn't used to getting this kind of attention. The main thing I was used to getting attention for was being cute. Anyway, under the tutelage of the English comp teacher, I was able to put together material for a biography on my grandmother, who published over fifty books. Most of them were about cowboys, or boys, since books about girls doing things didn't really sell in the sixties and seventies. I also started a play about her life. She was the first of ten children to break away from a Kansas wheat farm and go off to college. Later on, she became a teacher, and then, as I previously mentioned, an author. You would think with a grandmother who provided such a positive role model that I might not have gotten so sidetracked, but as you can see, I did.

And yet my grandmother did plant the seed. She helped me see that if you had a dream, eventually you could make it happen. In my case, the drugs and the alcohol that I began consuming at an early age made it next to impossible for me to consistently focus on my goals and dreams. The real me got covered up.

Anyway, when I got into the computer industry, a fledgling playwright and novelist, and third-generation writer (not to mention ex-call girl), I was definitely your proverbial fish out of water. Creative talent was, in the computer industry, a liability, not an asset. I was expected to edit and write highly technical instructional materials—nothing more, nothing less. No one wanted to hear about my brilliant marketing ideas, or my ideas for a novel, and so I learned quickly to hide my creative side—which is never a healthy thing to do.

When I entered the computer industry, we were still in what was called, "The Cold War." Each country felt they were the real superpower. Each country was highly suspicious of how the other side might be stockpiling nuclear arms and missiles. Many of the jobs that I held as a technical writer supported government and military efforts. On a few occasions I even had to obtain a top-secret clearance.

So I would sit there in my appropriate business attire and read top-secret documents about missile detection systems. And I would wonder when everyone would figure out I was an impostor—an alien creature—a non-technical woman. In other words, I was in over my head. In fact, things weren't going so well for me in the corporate world. I was so defensive, and so afraid people would find out who I really was, or worse yet, who I once had been.

I would hide whatever novel I was trying to write underneath the computer instructional manual I was editing. I had always wanted to be a novelist, just like my father. When my father wasn't locked up, there was always some book he was trying to write. Once he even claimed that a famous Hollywood screenwriter wanted to interview him and use his story in a movie about prison life. I guess eventually a film did get made, and one time, when my father got out of the "joint," he was short on what they call "gate money" (the cash given to convicts upon their release). Anyway, he said he wanted to find that director and screenwriter who had used his story and see if he could make some money. Like many things my father was involved in, nothing ever really panned out.

In addition to my secret career as an aspiring novelist, I really believed I had to be superwoman. The superwoman myth was big in the eighties. In a nutshell, this particular myth had more to do with acting like a man than anything else. A superwoman wore asexual haircuts, shoulder pads, had it all, did it all, and rejected anything feminine. Determined to prove that I was a superwoman in what was still a predominantly male workforce, I fought to climb the corporate ladder. I started off as a proofreader, became an editor, proceeded on as a jr. technical writer, then became a technical writer, and finally a technical trainer.

As I climbed that corporate ladder, my chief obstacle was not other employees—it was me. My alcoholism and drug addiction were progressing. When I was about 25, in 1984, I had a job as a technical writer and trainer at a software company in San Diego. I had been sent out of town to train at a Navy base. I had to stand up in front of a classroom, which at the time was highly embarrassing, since as a result of my cocaine addiction, I had a rash that formed a large circle underneath my nose. Up until I got this allergic reaction to cocaine, I had found it to be a useful numbing agent, in particular, with regard to freezing painful emotions. I had to go to a doctor about the rash, and I remember he asked me if I had a drug problem. "Of course not," I assured the skeptical doctor.

I was fired shortly after that. The company said I had too many mood swings, which were of course a direct result of my drug use. As my disease progressed, so did Craig's, who along with being an alcoholic and an addict also had a gambling problem.

One day, fed up with having to once again figure out how I'd be able to cover the never ending relentless flow of bad checks Craig had accrued in order to keep his gambling addiction going, I ran off with a black used car salesmen who I met at a bar. He provided me with an endless supply of cocaine to keep my addictions satisfied. Four days later, I returned home to Craig. The next week, I was served with divorce papers at my current place of employment, a computer company in San Diego.

From then on, not only was I, according to Craig, a whore, but I was also a "nigger-loving" whore. Domestic violence became a cornerstone to our relationship. To escape from my troubled marriage, I would often hit the singles bars…"meat markets"…and dance to Madonna, Michael Jackson, Depeche Mode, and of course, The Boss, Bruce Springsteen. Being that it was the eighties, we were into eighties styles, the music, the big hair…The only problem with me going to hang out at the singles bars was that …well…I had a tendency to drink those eighties style drinks in them: Kamikazes, Long Island Ice Teas. And whenever I drank alcohol, I could never be sure of what could, or would, happen next. Sometimes…many times…I wouldn't make it home. Needless to say this doesn't go over very well when you have a husband waiting for you.

Often I'd wind up in an alcoholic black out and when that happened too often I would end up consorting with men who then sometimes followed me into my *real* life. They would show up at my home, the one I shared with my husband. Or maybe drop in at my place of work. It was very difficult, constantly making up stories and lies, in order to explain this latest strange man to my husband, or latest employer. I often wouldn't even recognize the person I'd find before me. So in addition to my problems stemming from alcohol, party drugs, cocaine etc., I also had *another* underlying problem—I must have some kind of addiction to acting out sexually. Why else would I call myself the "single most married woman there ever was?"

Although my participation in the sex industry did not really include pornography, most of the sex I was having during the eighties was based on x-rated movies I had seen. These were movies with veteran porn stars such as Marilyn Chambers or Linda Lovelace, the star of that blockbuster *Deep Throat*, which brought XXX porn into the mainstream. Once VCRs became common household items of the eighties, movies like *Deep Throat* floated around in most people's homes.

These movies had a tremendous impact on what were my *already* impaired beliefs about what I thought it meant to be a sexual woman. In these movies, men must have endless erections and women were dumb whores that couldn't get enough. This seemed to become the status quo.

I believe what happened is that the pornographers exploited the masses, who, swept away with the glamour associated with men like Hugh Hefner the creator of *Playboy* magazine, wanted to claim that they too were sexually liberated, participants in the "sexual revolution." Thus greedy pornographers dictated a paradigm that promoted sexual behaviors based on prostitution, and was fueled by the success of movies like *Deep Throat*.

In other words, the sexual act had to be larger than life, a performance complete with lights, camera, action. It was all about acting like I couldn't get enough, like I was *Insatiable*, just like the title of the Marilyn Chambers XXX-rated movie. And although I was no longer turning tricks, all of my so-called romances were in fact based on drugs. If you had cocaine, I was in love. Give me enough cocaine and champagne, and I became an instant porn star, performing just for you. The only problem was the morning after, when I would have to deal with the two strangers before me— the stranger laying beside me, and my own reflection in the mirror.

While it was true that I was no longer in the sex industry, I was still acting out. I was completely ignorant to the fact that my need to act out sexually might indicate that I still had unresolved issues. And even if I did have a clue, I wouldn't have known how to identify, or what to call my problems. I did not have the words, the language to describe my still active addictions.

During the eighties, now in my twenties, I believed that I *had* to be sexual. Constantly. And so I would have affair after affair, repeatedly acting out the sexual trauma of my past. I was caught up in a spiral of shame; I was powerless. When I was sexually acting out, I became "the badgirl." In this persona, I became the ultimate whore who craved sex and the femme fatale who would not, *could* not be hurt. In alcoholic blackouts, I abandoned my marriage at every opportunity.

In reaction to my constant indiscretions, and total disregard to any fidelity, my husband Craig became increasingly violent towards me, and I guess I felt that I deserved it. In addition to his fury and rage over having a promiscuous wife, he would also criticize just about anything I did. He hated my cooking and felt I would purposefully ruin the laundry. So, feeling desperate to do what I could to save what was still left of my marriage, I tried using sex to "fix" the marriage. I felt like I was turning a trick.

My classy marriage may have been on the road to ruin due to my acting out, but at least I chose not to go find a madam, or a pimp, and I wasn't working as a prostitute…I mean call girl anymore. Besides, that had been a different me, a former life. My first husband and I lived in a beautiful home with a great view, and I still wanted desperately to believe that by leaving Baltimore and getting married, my past would be wiped out for good. I still attempted to sweep it all underground. Wasn't I now a good girl? Yet?

I've heard it said that "whoever you are follows you wherever you go," and even though I wasn't officially in the sex industry anymore, or selling or "renting" myself sexually to whoever had enough money, I still was engaged in the sale of my sex, the only difference being that instead of charging a flat fee, I received the security, power and freedom to live a "charmed life." The cost to my soul was much greater.

The first marriage to that Prince Charming lasted only until 1985, when the Major asked us to move out of the palace. Craig filed for a divorce for the second, and final time. Newly separated from Craig, I moved to a great apartment in downtown San Diego, which I paid for through my work as a technical editor at yet another computer company. The apartment had a fantastic view of the harbor and city skyline, but I might as well have been looking at a brick wall. Since my alcoholism was progressing at an alarming rate, I really couldn't enjoy San Diego's beauty.

All I knew is that I wanted…now I *needed*…the next drink, or pill, or line of coke so that I would not have to feel any pain resulting from my soon to be coming divorce, or long buried memories of the past. I prided myself on being able to hook up with drug dealers so that I could get my drugs for free, or at least at a reduced cost. *Sex in exchange for drugs. There's nothing wrong with that,* I reassured myself. Whenever my emotions about my failed marriage would flare up, I'd call up one of those dealers.

But drugs and alcohol couldn't satisfy my craving for the next relationship, so I constantly went from man to man. I began to develop a nasty reputation in the bars I frequented. Men started to reject me on a regular basis. Much to my own shock and dismay, they actually felt I was too wild.

But where the opposite sex was concerned, I always had a backup plan, or a private stash, so to speak. Just like alcoholics keep a bottle hidden "just in case," I had my New York City man, D.H. When I was between marriages, or my attempts at relationships, I would fly to New York. I met D.H. for the first time months before the end of my first marriage. He had handed me a vile of cocaine and it was love at first blast.

It was a long-distance, chemically based romance. But no matter how big the piles of cocaine, or how long the lines were, it was never enough. No matter how much I drank, snorted or smoked, I could never find the right combination. I flew back and forth between the East Coast and the West Coast, just as I had done my entire life, on the run from a storm of emotions buried deep inside.

Spring, 1986
Hitting Bottom

And then I met Armando, a perfect mirror for my diseased, addicted self. Armando claimed he was in the Portuguese Mafia. For the most part, Armando was really just a drug dealer. For a few weeks, I felt like I had hit the boyfriend jackpot. But quickly enough, my relationship with him became extremely painful. And even though he always supplied me with the best in designer drugs and the finest wines and champagnes, it was never enough.

Despite the fact that I had a good job and a nice apartment, something was not quite right. For one thing, I didn't like the kind of woman I felt I was becoming again. I felt shattered, not whole, and desperate to fix myself from the outside. Who I was, and who I had been in my past, nipped at my heals, like the tornado chasing Dorothy in the "Wizard of Oz."

The tools that I had used to survive in the sex industry, such as running away, shutting down, and drugs and alcohol, weren't working in the new world I inhabited. Sometimes I would wake up still clenching a cigarette I'd been smoking the night before, and I didn't even consider myself a smoker. Once again, who I was on the outside clashed with who I believed myself to be on the inside.

One day, I walked down the strip of beach that was right outside of Armando's apartment. I had spent the night with him. All night long, a parade of drug addicts came in to get their supply of cocaine and crystal meth. I would wait in the corner for my supply of both chemicals, and something else—Armando's love and attention. Since Armando was both a drug addict and a sex addict, and I was just one of the many names he kept in his gold-plated rolodex, sometimes I waited a long, long time.

As I walked along the water's edge, watching the surf move in and out, I thought about the latest piece of jewelry that Armando had promised me, and tried to convince myself that as soon as he gave it to me, I would feel complete.

But something in me knew that I was lying to myself, and I began to feel a sense of hopelessness. I had never felt so alone in my entire life. Usually some combination of these three items (men, drugs, or alcohol) numbed the pain I sought so desperately to run from, but not anymore. I did not know that I was hitting bottom. I did not know then that I was spiritually bankrupt. As I peered at the shimmering Pacific Ocean, I wondered, *did I scratch and crawl out of the sex industry to wind up living like this?*

A woman named Sandy moved into my downtown San Diego apartment who was clean and sober. Sandy brought it to my attention that by constantly focusing on men, I was missing the opportunity to find out who I really was. Sandy had dated many famous powerful men, including Elvis and Ted Turner.

One day, the two of us were having one of the open, honest discussions typical of our deepening friendship. "I dated womanizers," Sandy said. "Men who had many other women in their lives. I did everything I could to be the perfect woman for them, and I lost myself in the process."

Sandy, who was seventeen years older than me, admitted to having an addiction to love. She told me about something called codependency, which she said was an inability to set appropriate boundaries. I felt as if I was learning a new language.

I was able to talk to her with an honesty that was new to me. And she listened. But I never told her about my past. I was too ashamed. How could a nice girl like me, with a college degree, working as a technical writer by day and as a novelist by night possibly have a past like that?

1987
San Diego, California

Sandy brought me to my first AA meeting in the spring of 87. It was Easter. For the first time in my entire life, I made a connection with the idea of a spiritual rebirth. A part of me, the alcoholic/addict aspect of myself, was dying so that my real, authentic self could be reborn.

My experience of being reborn was short lived however, and, after a few months of complete sobriety, I relapsed. I was invited to go see a Madonna concert. Someone brought out some cocaine, and I convinced myself that I would just do it this one last time.

After I used, I tried to convince myself I hadn't really relapsed because I didn't consume alcohol.

Continuing along with my mental gymnastics, I adroitly reasoned that since I had already used the cocaine, I might as well go to a place where there would be unlimited supplies for a discounted rate. Within 24 hours, I was on a plane headed for New York to visit my rainy-day man, D.H. I white-knuckled it the entire time on the plane ride, refusing any drinks that the flight attendants kept offering me.

But the obsession was already in place, and as soon as I got into the city, I found myself on a barstool staring down an exotic frozen beverage complete with a cute little paper umbrella floating at the top. As I drank that first drink—a pina colada—I had this awful, out of control feeling. It was similar to losing your virginity, too soon, to the wrong person. I began to understand that I really did have a problem. I watched myself drink and use. Night after night, while my friend D.H. slept, I was on the hunt for more drugs.

But no matter how much I was able to find and consume, it was never enough. After doing about two weeks of research, in August of 1987, I dragged myself back into the rooms of Alcoholics Anonymous. Both strung out and hung over, I slumped down into my chair, completely defeated yet somehow at peace. I was beginning to surrender.

I met husband-to-be number two in an AA meeting when I was only one month sober. Once again, I cast a man who I hardly knew in the role of protector and savior. Only months into a legal separation with my first husband, I went from the frying pan right into the fire with my next relationship. I was, after all, highly skilled in ignoring red flags that indicate a volatile, abusive temperament.

I had a habit of picking angry, abusive and controlling men who reinforced my sense of worthlessness. And Patrick fit the bill perfectly. I looked across the smoky Alano club, and I thought; now that guy looks angry. Every time he raged, I made excuses for his behavior, and I wished it away. It was only because he was newly sober, or because he was having trouble finding a job.

To make this relationship even more challenging, Patrick was a member of the burgeoning Christian Right. Because of his beliefs, he resented the fact that I had an abortion on two occasions. Patrick believed that abortion was murder. To make matters worse, he was a terrible bigot, so the fact that I had been with lovers of ethnic backgrounds other than white made his blood boil.

I didn't want to face the truth about his rage, because then I might have to stop and deal with some unfinished business. Like the painful dissolution of my first marriage, and my years as a sex worker. Despite all the red flags, and all the obvious differences in our personalities, I turned a deaf ear to the countless people who told me that it might be best if I at least allowed the ink to dry on my divorce papers before I rushed into this relationship.

chapter fourteen

Back to the Nineties
San Diego

When I was in the sex industry, I never had an official pimp. But psychologically, the men I chose post sex industry were similar to pimps. Each one was controlling, punishing, and critical. Each one told me I was worthless, and I believed it. Each one made me feel that I would be nothing without their love.

And so desperate to attain this love, I attempted to mold myself into whatever it was that I thought they wanted me to be. Did they want me thin? Well, it must be time to diet and hit the gym. How about hair preference—did they want blonde, or brunette? My first husband wanted a brunette. I let my natural color grow out, but as soon as we separated, I became a blonde again.

Who did they want me to be? That was who I became, a perfect chameleon. I had the *Cosmopolitan* magazine inspired belief that if I shaped myself into the perfect feminine Barbie doll I would get love. As any Cosmo girls knows, you had to be sexual to get a man's love. The only problem with this is that the double standard that applied to female sexuality is still very much alive and well. We're basically talking about a no-win situation, you're damned if you do, damned if you don't type of thing. In essence, or to summarize, the double standard implies that while sexual men are heroes, a sexual woman is an evil, dangerous, life-sucking creature.

And since a sexual girl was a bad girl, I lived shrouded in shame, a shame that followed me wherever I went. I stood outside of myself, as if I was watching a movie about who I was. I was split. Not whole. The choices I made when I was a prostituted girlwoman still haunt me. My experiences as a prostituted woman have been lodged into my cells and into the blood that pumps through my body. The sex industry is lethal. It can destroy a person. I've seen it happen. It just about happened to me.

That I am still alive is a miracle. Participation in the sex industry is like walking around with a gun pointed to your head. At any moment, the gun might go off, and you could become another statistic. Just another Jane Doe. But when you are in it, you really are not dealing with reality.

You know the danger is real, but, like everything else, to survive in that world, you have to shut out the truth. Because deep down you don't really think you are "that kind of a girl." Even though I wasn't officially in the industry any longer, I still had not healed the whoregirl inside. There was a terrible emptiness in me that even my sobriety in Alcoholics Anonymous could not address.

What I went through scarred me and hurt me in a way that can never be completely healed. And yet I had to attempt to make peace with my past, or forever recreate it. And although I had been out of the sex industry for over a decade, and even though I was clean and sober, I still did things that reminded me of the little lost hooker girl.

I knew that true healing would never come for me until I could bring the dark storm of my past out into the light. I never thought

I would be able to talk about what really happened, about the days and nights in Baltimore when I had played the whore to countless strangers. And maybe I never would have, if I hadn't run into Denise again.

* * *

August 1991
Pacific Beach Alano Club, San Diego

"I came to in jail and I looked around," she said, in the blackest white girl accent I had ever heard. "And once I realized where I was, I thought, 'what the hell am I doing here?' I remember thinking, 'Well, shit, at least I must look better than the rest of these raggedy bitches.' At that time I was practically hairless and I weighed less than ninety pounds soaking wet. What happened to me is that my alcoholism and drug addiction led me into prostitution, which naturally, led me into getting locked up in jail."

You could hear a pin drop! As I glanced around the crowded AA meeting hall, I checked to see how others might be responding. No one seemed as shocked as I was. I couldn't *believe* she had actually said it! She had said the dirty "P" word. I felt horrified for her, as if she had just paraded around the room naked. "She" was Denise—the woman from the Sex and Love Addicts Anonymous meeting. It was a Friday night, and I had walked into the meeting alone. I was supposed to meet Patrick here, and quite frankly, I was elated he hadn't shown up yet. Had he been here listening, he would have been horrified by what Denise had just said.

After the meeting closed, I approached her and said, "Hi, it's me, Juliet. Do you remember me?"

"Of course I remember you Juliet," she responded, giving me a warm hug.

"You sure are honest, Denise."

"Thanks," she said, pushing her hair behind her. "It's either that or drink again. That's why I joined a group called Sex Industry Survivors Anonymous."

I just stared at her. Surely there must be something wrong with this wild-eyed, frizzy-haired person. Not only was she admitting to her past, but she was also admitting to being involved in a group called Sex Industry Survivors Anonymous.

"I've been out of all that for a few months now," she said. "It really helps to talk about it."

She looked at me an extra few seconds and as I noticed how very blue her eyes were, I heard a tiny voice, my *own*, saying: "I was into all that."

She then broke into a smile, gave me a hug, and asked, "Would you like to come to our group sometime?"

"Oh, no thanks!" I said, backing away from her. "I'm just trying to get the AA thing down right now; you know what I mean?"

"Yeah, I do know what you mean."

"Thanks, and hey it was nice seeing you again." I started to walk away and just when I thought I had made a clean getaway I heard her calling my name.

"Juliet!"

I turned around to face her. "Yes?"

"Are you sure?"

"Excuse me?"

"What I mean is, why can't you come check it out, just one time?"

"But I've never talked about…*that* before," I said.

"Then you need to," Denise said. "*Especially* if you want to stay sober. Those secrets will get you drunk—you know what I mean homegirl?"

"I guess it couldn't hurt," I said. As I felt my fear breaking down, I broke into a smile.

"You go girl; *two snaps up*. One thing though—I'm glad I remembered—we'll have to get you cleared first."

"*Cleared?*"

"Yeah, cleared, through the San Diego Sheriff's Department. The meeting is in the Los Colinas Women's Jail, down in Santee. I'm certain you'll have no problem getting cleared."

"I think I've heard of it," I said, clearing my throat.

The truth was, not only had I *heard* of it, but I had actually spent a few hours in a holding cell there, back when *I* was arrested by the San Diego Sheriffs, for drunk driving. Since that incident had been well over seven years ago, I was pretty sure it wouldn't show up on my record, and that Denise was probably correct in assuming I'd be approved.

I was quite intoxicated at the time of my arrest, just a week before Thanksgiving, in 1983. I had been drinking heavily and snorting lines of meth for several hours that particular night. This combination can be deceptively dangerous, in that the speed would seem to hide my sense of alcoholic intoxication while at the same time creating a ludicrous sense of what I perceived as my own invincibility. Indeed, I might have *thought* I was superwoman, but, upon receiving the sobriety tests, I could not walk a straight line, nor could I even recite the alphabet backward or forward.

But that did nothing to inhibit me from trying to work those cops to change their minds and let me go. "Just let me drive home," I pleaded, "I'm almost there, please..."

"Aren't they all," said one of the cops, who, to my chagrin, chose to not only deny my simple, reasonable request to drive home—*he* drove me—to Santee, instead of taking me home to pass out in my own bed.

At the time, although my blood alcohol level really had been dangerously high, I really and truly resented the fact that they had pulled a *nice girl like me* over! I tried everything in my power to fight the charges by hiring an expensive lawyer, who, in the end, managed to do absolutely nothing for me. I remember standing in front of the judge who asked me "Had you been drinking when you were arrested?"

"Yes," I mumbled. For reasons I'd yet to fully comprehend I remember feeling stunned when, even after retaining a "fixit" lawyer, I was still charged with driving under the influence. I was still a long, long way from recognizing that I had the disease of alcoholism.

September 1991
Los Colinas Women's Jail
Santee, California

It took roughly a month for the Sheriff's department to check me out, clear me, and then one bright sunny day, I returned to the dull, gray institution, where I had previously been a guest. Upon arrival, I pulled my white 1988 Firebird Pontiac into the parking lot of the women's jail. Then, only a few minutes later, a beat-up Chevy Impala entered the parking lot and parked in the space right next to mine.

I watched Denise and a dark-haired, abundantly sized woman who wore very baggy clothing get out of the car and walk towards me. "This is Joanne," Denise said excitedly. "She's the founder of Sex Industry Survivors Anonymous."

"I'm glad to meet you, Joanne. I'm Juliet," I said, extending my hand. "I've never met the founder of anything before."

"Well you have now," Joanne said, smiling.

Looking at Joanne, I decided she should definitely do something about her hair and clothes. But I soon learned that there was a reason for her plain Jane appearance.

"I know my way around pretty well," Denise said. "I was a guest here on many occasions. Now, the beauty is that I get to leave."

I knew from following my convict dad from institution to institution that being able to leave was definitely a plus, but I didn't respond to her comment. At the front entrance of the jail, a clerk looked our names up and then admitted us into a tiny room adjacent to the reception area. Just for a moment, the doors automatically slid shut. I felt claustrophobic—what if the didn't let us out? Finally, one by one, we were admitted into a holding area.

"Betty Broderick was just in here," Denise said. Betty Broderick was on trial for murdering her ex-husband and his new wife while they slept.

Hell hath no fury like a woman scorned, I thought, as we followed the deputy through the bowels of the gray institution. If you have ever had the misfortune to be inside a jail you know that there is an aroma that could only be called eau de Jail. The scent, a mix between antiseptic cleaners, perspiration, and human beings in captivity, is really quite sad.

Inmates sat on a bench in a holding tank room. Waiting.

Years ago, I sat on that very bench, wondering how they could possibly have arrested a nice girl like me. But they *had* arrested me, and they had arrested these women, and now some of them glanced furtively through the smudged plastic window in the holding tank, their eyes desperate, pleading. I found it impossible to make eye contact, and suddenly I was overcome with guilt because I was not a prisoner like them.

Inmates dressed in paper-thin blue uniforms moved slowly down the too-narrow halls. Inmates working in the laundry room peered at us as we walked past them. Others, their hair confined in standard issue plastic bonnets, paid us no mind and focused instead on folding white sheet after white sheet. In a less than spacious recreation-type room prisoners stared at an episode of Oprah, hypnotized.

The walls seemed to press in closer, and the eau de jail aroma hovered around us, thick, miasmic. The deputy led us into a small room that had been set up like a classroom. The three of us sat in the front of a table that faced out towards the rows of desks. After about ten minutes a female deputy sheriff lead a small group of women into our classroom. Three were black, two Hispanic, and one was white.

"We would have had more inmates but they were embarrassed," explained a woman wearing a plastic jail employee badge that read: "Doreen, Counselor."

"Hey Doreen, that's okay," said Denise. "No problem. Doreen, this is Joanne, and Juliet."

"Glad to meet both of you. The women have been looking forward to this."

The women, shifting uncomfortably in their seats, didn't look like they were looking forward to this very much at all.

"We better get started," Denise said to Joanne.

Joanne nodded and started the meeting. "I'm Joanne, and I'm a recovering prostitute. I sent an article around that describes how I used to be, so that you can all see the extremes we can bounce back from. As you can tell from the article, the escort service I ran with my mother was so notorious that we both made the news. But even after we got closed down, I continued, this time not as a madam, but as a prostitute. I would try and start regular jobs but managers from the escort service would find ways to get me fired so that I would have to go back to work for them.

"When I finally turned my first trick there were two of them—one was waiting in the closet—and one was ready to beat me up if I didn't do both of them. I ran, and they chased after me, and I remember thinking, *'Boy, this is neat.'* And so the addiction began. It was an addiction to adrenaline. I would always take on the dangerous customers because I felt most alive with them."

The women are spellbound. Denise is busy chomping gum. It's really starting to irritate me. I keep glancing over at her, thinking that maybe she'll catch the hint, and stop chewing it, but she doesn't. I wasn't sure what kind of example we were setting with her chewing gum like that.

"I tried all different ways of living the life," Joanne went on. "I tried being a madam, I tried phone sex, I tried all aspects of the sex industry. I became addicted to the money. I even realize now that I actually had blackouts in the disease, just like an alcoholic."

As I sat in my plastic chair in the makeshift classroom, I didn't feel comfortable, not one bit, no matter how many different positions I sat in. Besides, I was nothing like this woman. I hadn't gone down as far as she did. But then, out of nowhere, I was struck with a more enlightened thought.

Maybe I wasn't so different from Joanne, and maybe I wasn't so different from these incarcerated women. The only real difference between me and them was that I had never gotten arrested, at least not for prostitution. My new insight helped me relax a little bit, and finally finding comfort in the orange plastic chair, I turned my attention back to Joanne.

"When I found out about twelve-step programs I was afraid; I didn't know if I would fit in," Joanne admitted. "The women in other groups were offended when I talked about prostitution. But that had been my life. I wore spandex pants and big gaudy rings. People looked at me like I was a freak.

"Finally, I asked this guy to be my sponsor. The first thing he did was tell me to lose the spandex." The women thought that was hilarious. "Next, he made me cut off my long, blonde hair. He said it was a walking advertisement. The day I got my hair cut, I cried as I watched it fall to the ground. But I also knew I didn't have a choice anymore. The disease of addiction was killing me. I was addicted to prostitution."

The women peered at us, almost looking a little interested. *So that was the reason for the plain Jane look,* I thought.

"It ain't no such thing as an addiction," contested a toothless black woman. "I do it so I can get my crack."

Undaunted, Joanne went on. "I understand—many of us have multiple addictions. And the statistics are out. If you are both an alcoholic *and* an addict, as well as being a victim of child abuse or prostitution, the statistics say you have a 95 percent mortality rate. Quite simply our disease wants to kill us."

Her grim statistics shot a bolt of white fear through me. I always knew I had been lucky to be alive, but until *now,* I had no idea just *how* lucky.

"Shit," piped up the black woman again. "You can drive in your car one day an' git' killed—t'aint no big thing."

Joanne just shook her head. "Believe it or not, prostitution is not just something women do to support a drug habit. I know a woman who was making over sixty thousand a year in advertising who went back into the life. It's an addiction. It's an addiction to the sex industry. Today I am not acting out in any way. I only work this one program, Sex Industry Survivors Anonymous, and I have a female sponsor. I'm married and I have a child. When you stop acting out in any way you get a real clean connection with your higher power. My direct link told me to get married and have my child."

"Juliet, would you like to share with the group?" Denise asked.

"I'm Juliet," I said tentatively. "And I'm a recovering call girl."

"Hi Juliet," the panel leaders chimed in unison.

"Hi," I said. "I'm glad to be here, but I have to admit, I'm scared. I've never talked about any of this before. It's hard for me to say that word…prostitution. I always tried to just say I was a call girl, because I thought that made what I was doing sound more glamorous."

Just then, I felt my throat closing up. An ancient pain was erupting, and I could not go on. Instead, I gazed up at the huge clock facing me. Even though I could see, and hear, that seconds were clicking past, it seemed as if time had stopped. A couple of the women coughed, nervous, shifting in their seats.

"It's okay, Juliet," Joanne said sympathetically, bringing me back into the moment, "You can call it whatever you want."

"Yeah, well, I've kept all this a secret for ten years so it isn't going to be easy for me to talk about it." Joanne and Denise looked over at me, and somehow their presence was reassuring.

"Anyway, I really wasn't a prostitute," I explained. "I was a call girl. I led a double life. I wanted to take from all men. I thought they all owed me something. Maybe I hated them, I don't know. My father was never there for me so I knew I was always on my own. I was terrified at times about how I would get by. And so I got into prostitution.

"I remember this client took me out for dinner. I was trying to run this game on him—I wanted him to be a sugar daddy, you know, take care of me. As it turned out, he refused. He was almost seventy, and he already had a 27-year-old mistress. He owned all these strip clubs in the red light section of Baltimore. Like he couldn't have afforded two women. That still pisses me off to this day."

"Oh, you know it, girlfriend got played by the player," chimed in the toothless black woman. Everyone just cracked up at that.

"The guy that I was trying to con into setting me up took me downtown to the Holiday Inn in Baltimore. I begged him to reconsider my offer. I remember thinking, I'm only 21, and he should want me. I was pissed. After he was done, I was trying to call all these other guys, you know, to get the next client lined up. I kept calling and calling—I was desperate. I just had to get the *next* customer over there.

"Looking back, that's one of the clearest examples of how my addiction to the sex industry progressed. It wasn't something I had any control over anymore. I was locked into that behavior, or compulsion, whatever you want to call it. It wasn't enough to turn a trick. I had to manipulate, con the trick into agreeing to be my sugar daddy. And one sugar daddy wouldn't be enough. Since I was earning money to pay for my college tuition through turning tricks, I used to always tell myself, I'll just do it one more semester, and then I'll quit. But I never did.

"Joanne says it's an addiction to the sex industry, so maybe that's what it was. And that night at that Holiday Inn my addiction seemed to have gone into some sort of progression. I was hitting a bottom, crossing all kinds of boundaries I never thought I would.

"That was 10 years ago," I heard myself saying to the women in the jail classroom. "I'm 31 now. I left that life behind ten years ago when I flew 3,000 miles to marry my first husband."

The pain started coalescing in my throat again, and the room felt like it was closing in on me. The inmates peered at me, curious.

"I thought I could just leave everything behind but I guess it doesn't work that way. Now I'm divorced from my first husband and I'm about to marry my second husband. Sometimes I wonder if I've changed at all. I get these obsessions of the mind where I want to use men, just like in my past. For example, I was having an affair with someone, and I ended it when I met someone who I thought might be wealthy. So I told him I was unbelievable in bed. I worked that angle for a while, but he figured out pretty quickly what I was up to. I can't play the game anymore. Actually, I never could to begin with. I see myself as a sort of failed hooker."

"Failed hooker," laughed a black girl. "Ain't that some shit. My name Lateshia."

"Hi Lateshia," the members of the group replied back.

"I thought you said you was engaged," Lateshia said. "Do he

know you was a ho'?"

"Ugh, no, no he doesn't," I mumbled.

"Why he not know, how come you ain't tol' him?"

I had no answer for her.

"My name is Denise and I am a recovering hooker. I started when I was 18. I was a virgin and I had never even had sex before. He took me to a cemetery. He told me to suck his cock and I did. Then I watched him jerk himself off. He gave me twenty dollars. After I did that, I felt like such a tramp. I wondered how I could do such an awful thing.

"Then I met this terrible man, who wanted me to do all nude dancing. I wouldn't do it, but I needed to get away from my father, because he was so crazy. So I did a geographic. I got on a bus and moved to California.

"I began to prostitute myself on the streets on a daily basis. I was addicted to heroin—yes. But that wasn't why I was a prostitute. I loved the excitement, the danger. I was addicted to the power and I loved being in control. It was also all about revenge. Every trick I turned was revenge on my father since he was so abusive. Once he turned on an iron and began to iron my arm. I still have scars from that.

"You see, every time I turned a trick, I died a little more inside. Every time I gave my body away, there was a little less of me inside. And that's why I did it. Because I hated myself."

And so we three women on the newly formed ladies-of-the night panel had all talked about what had happened to us. And the women in the dubious classroom looked back at us. Some were young, but most, despite their chronological age, looked tired, and battle-scarred.

chapter fifteen

"You look like you're about to faint," Denise said.

I was giving her a ride home after the meeting at Los Colinas Women's Jail. "I'm fine," I said, my voice breaking up a little.

"You don't sound fine."

"Like I said, I'm fine."

"Well then how come you look like you're about to cry?" She asked.

I pulled the rear-view mirror down and checked myself out. "I look okay."

"You really haven't talked about this stuff before, have you?"

I shook my head. "No, I haven't, and if Patrick finds out, the wedding will be cancelled."

"Well, if you can't tell him who you really are, maybe that's not such a bad thing." She paused and then said, "Has it occurred to you that maybe you're rushing into this marriage? Maybe you should wait a while."

I looked at Denise like she was crazy. *Wait* to get married? Why would I do that? I needed a man to take care of me. Yes, I was a trained professional, a technical writer employed in the computer industry. But in terms of survival, I had it hard wired into my brain that it would be best if a man were to rush in at the last minute and come to my rescue. And so I was annoyed by her suggestion that I might be rushing into this marriage.

I simply had to be married. Marriage represented security to me, and I was addicted to security. "I'm in love," I contested. "Why should I wait to get married?"

"Well, to begin with, you're afraid to tell him about your past," Denise said. "Isn't that going to create problems down the road?"

We were leaving the strip malls and country western Dive bars of Santee. "I don't know. I'm just not ready to say anything right now."

"But you've been out of it for a long time now."

"Have I? Sometimes I'm not so sure," I said softly. "I mean, I'm not turning tricks anymore, but I have this secret life going on behind Patrick's back."

"That all may be true, but you aren't in the sex industry anymore."

"Yes, and no," I muttered.

"Girl, what are you talking about?"

"I'm not sure if you really *can* leave the sex industry behind—not completely anyway. It's like you're branded…like you've got this tattoo on your soul."

"You aren't doing what you used to do, right?"

"No," I admitted, "I'm not. "But I just shared something I thought I would take to the grave with me. And I shared it with a bunch of locked up women who looked like they saw right through me."

"What are you taking about?" Denise said.

I sighed. "I felt like a phony. I said I was out of all of it, but sometimes I wonder if I really have changed, or if I'm—"

"Damaged goods?" Denise said.

"Yeah, something like that," I said, and turned my Pontiac onto the exit marked San Diego.

Denise and I were walking through the courtyard that led to my condo. I had talked her into coming over for a while.

"You know there may be an opportunity for us to get on the news," she said.

"Why would we want to go on the news?" I asked, as I turned the key to the front door and let us both in.

"To spread the word. There's this reporter from the *San Diego Sun* who wants our story. And Joanne wants us to go on the Oprah show."

"The Oprah Winfrey show?"

"The one and only," Denise confirmed, depositing herself on my living room couch. "We would be representing Sex Industry Survivors Anonymous."

I took a seat next to her on the couch. "Wouldn't that be something. With my luck, on my honeymoon night, my new hubby would turn the TV on, and there I'd be, donning a wig and sunglasses."

Denise laughed. "If you had a disguise on he wouldn't recognize you."

"Right," I said, shaking my head. "What would that little caption underneath me say? 'ENGAGED WOMAN REVEALS SECRET PAST'…"

She shrugged her shoulders. "Or you could have it say: 'ENGAGED WOMAN TELLS THE MAN SHE IS ABOUT TO MARRY THAT SHE WAS A HO'."

"Yeah, that's even better," I had to admit. "Look, are you really considering going on national television?"

"I want to do it, but…"

"But what?" I asked.

"I'm not exactly sober," Denise said.

"What do you mean you're not sober? You mean from prostitution—not sober from prostitution?" She nodded. "I thought you said in the jail just now that you had been out of it for a few months."

"About two weeks ago I called an escort service. I did an in-call. All I did was dance for him, but I'm telling you, just doing that triggered my addiction. Now I can't stop thinking about the next client."

"What do you mean, you wanna go turn tricks or something?" I asked.

She nodded.

"It really is an addiction, isn't it?" I said. "Like drinking that first drink. But what's the first drink in this addiction?"

"The first transaction. And see, even though I didn't turn an official trick—I didn't have sex with the guy—I know it was a transaction, an exchange. And once I started thinking about calling the escort service, I felt like I had no choice. I just had to do it, and it isn't like I need the money. I have a job as an accountant, and I'm married."

"If you didn't need the money then why did you do it?"

"I just couldn't get the thought out of my mind, and then I acted on it. Even though I had that slip, well, I know that I've gotten better. Hell, back in the day, I was stripping, hooking, and acting in porn. In fact, the guy that I did the in-call with remembered me from one of my movies."

My jaw dropped. "Your movies—you were in movies?"

"I've been in about 400 movies."

"What kind of movies?" I asked, as if I didn't know.

"Porno."

"400 movies?" I stammered, absolutely dumfounded.

"Give or take a few."

Graphic images snaked through my mind, a cesspool of faceless bodies pressed together; anonymous, meaningless, loveless. As usual, when I thought of the sex industry, I experienced both revulsion *and* fascination.

Then I remembered that day in Baltimore; I was about eighteen. A dark sedan pulled up and the tinted car window floated down. "Hey sweetheart," said the stranger in the sedan. "Do you want to be an actress? Do you want to be our next porn star?" I ran away and I could hear the man who had propositioned me laughing…

"Hey, what's wrong, cat got your tongue," Denise said, as she trailed a finger along my cheekbone.

"Don't!" I warned, pulling away from her.

"What were you thinking about just then Juliet; you went into another world. Were you thinking about me in all those movies?"

"No, what you told me triggered this memory of when I was about eighteen and this guy asked me if I wanted to be a porn star."

"And what if he could have made you a porn star—would you have liked it? All those cameras on you, all that power, all that money."

"Stop it," I snapped. "Of course I wouldn't have liked it. It's just another form of prostitution, Denise. Legalized prostitution. Paid rape with the camera roll—"

Denise cut me off mid-sentence with, "Paid rape, that's ridiculous…with the kind of money I made, I'd hardly be able to call it rape."

"Sexual exploitation packaged differently, that's all. In some ways, it's even more dangerous."

"Why is that?"

"Film lasts forever."

She smiled sweetly at me, as if I was a pathetic, naïve child, and came closer to me, too close, her demeanor becoming strangely seductive. "You're such a warrior; always ready to do battle. I'm just wondering…does the idea that I was in all those movies disgust you, or does it turn you on?"

She laughed, and it made a chill go through me. "You just really confuse me, you know that? It seems like you still miss that whole world. You do, don't you?"

"Some things about it, yeah, I guess I do. I miss the excitement, and sometimes I even miss the danger," Denise said, her blue eyes narrowing as she contemplated the world she couldn't seem to leave behind. "The only thing I don't miss is getting locked up."

"Yeah, it's strange, when I was into all that it never even crossed my mind that what I was doing was illegal."

"When they slam that jail cell door behind you, it'll come back to you, believe me," she said, grinning. "But I know what you mean."

I nodded, and all the talk of jails reminded me of my father, state raised by the California Department of Corrections. "When we went to the jail and had the meeting with the women it made me realize how lucky I was that *I* never got arrested. But there's a part of me that's doing the time anyway."

"What are you talking about?" Denise said.

"I still feel trapped by my past. I'm not free of it because I tried for over a decade to act like nothing happened. All that pain didn't go away just because I pretended it wasn't there." I shook my head, not really sure myself where I was going with all this. "The memories are like prison bars that hold me back from really living my life," I said, my voice quavering. "If that makes any sense."

Then I got up and went to the kitchen, stalling for time so I could find the words to articulate the cauldron of emotions, thoughts and memories exploding inside of me. I poured bottled water over ice into a tall glass. I carried my drink back into the living room. "Sometimes I think I blame myself for what I did. It's not like anyone put a gun to my head and forced me into prostitution. It's just so painful-healing from this."

Denise got up from the sofa. For some odd reason, just then we both ended up standing in front of large antique mirror that hung above the sofa.

"Look at us," I said. "Who are we really, don't you wonder?" Denise was looking at me like I was crazy, but I went on. "Maybe those women in jail have more integrity than I do. They say they don't know if they're ready to get out of it. At least that's honest. I say I'm out of it, but am I?"

"Girl, you're starting to scare me—you know that? You're supposed to be my pillar of strength, and here you are carrying on like this."

I sighed deeply. "I'm just a good actress...Sometimes at night I wake up in a cold sweat from a nightmare—another nightmare—some trick's face, and then the image morphs, changes into my stepfather's face. Next I often see huge bodies of water, or I think I might be drowning, and so I try to pull myself out of the dream. Have you ever had dreams like that?"

"Yes," she said simply, and once again our eyes met in the big mirror we were both facing, and for the first time since I had known her, I thought I saw tears in her eyes. We both sunk back into the couch and Denise continued with, "I've had horrible dreams, and devastating memories, but we're healing, aren't we? And things will get better. After all no matter what you say, you did get out. You got a job in the computer world. You're a professional, you are a survivor, Juliet."

"Thanks, Denise, I just wish I could really believe all that, but deep down I just feel like my life is a big lie. And my thinking is beginning to really scare me."

"Why does it scare you?" Denise asked.

"I feel like I'm right on that edge, like I'm right about to go back to my old ways," I replied. Then Denise put her arms around me and I felt the corners of my mouth pulling down and that old pain started up again and I said, as we gently moved apart again, "I just wish I never got into the sex industry. In so many ways it's ruined my life." A big fat tear threatened to spill down my cheek. The tear had a mind of its own; I brushed it away, impatient with my own humanity. "I just want this pain to go away."

"I know, honey, I know."

When I had been in the life, or the world of the sex industry, I never thought about the consequences. It never even crossed my mind that I was participating in criminal activities. And even though I escaped the legal repercussions associated with sex work, there were very significant consequences—psychological consequences—still facing me.

In short, I doubted my own integrity; that is if I ever had any. I had talked about my past in front of a group of incarcerated women. I said I was no longer in that lifestyle. But how much of that was true? I was still living a double life. I was having affair after affair, and I couldn't stop.

Later that evening, I asked Denise if she would go to Kix, the nightclub, with me.

"No, you can't go to Kix," she said.

"But I always go to Kix on Thursday nights," I explained.

Denise looked me square in the eyes. "You wanna go there when you're all messed up like this? You opened up Pandora's box, Juliet. You're talking about stuff you've never talked about before. It's obvious you're in a lot of pain."

"I'm fine, really. Besides, there's this guy I like. His name is Tony. I can't get him out of my mind."

"Doesn't it scare you that you're about to get married and you can't stop thinking about other guys?"

"I just have to get it out of my system," I rationalized. "It's like when I knew I was about to quit drinking, I went around with a drink in either hand—I couldn't get enough."

Denise nodded. "Since we're being so honest, there's something I need to tell you. I had another slip, other than the one I told you about."

"Another slip?" I said with complete disbelief.

"It was about a month ago. I went back down to the whore strip. I went back down to El Cajon Boulevard."

Once again, my jaw dropped. "You did what?"

"I went back to the ho' stro'—you know, the boulevard. Every town has a stroll."

I shook my head. "But I thought you said in the meeting that you'd been out of the sex industry for three months."

"I know I said that; yes, well, I felt I had to say that. I want those women to know there is hope, and—"

"Look," I cut in. "You don't have to explain to me why you lied. It's not like I'm your parole officer or anything."

"I know that," Denise responded. "I just want you to understand what happened—why I went back out there."

"I'm listening."

"I was having an anxiety attack."

"Why?"

"I had this panicky feeling, like something bad was going to go down with my marriage. My husband and I had been fighting. I just didn't feel like we could make it work, and so I found myself driving down to the stroll.

"At first I told myself that I was just going to say hello to some of my homegirls I've worked with over the years. I was planning on having a little fun and then I would just go home and make up with my husband. But as soon as I got down there I started to just get into the scene. I was getting a rush from all the excitement—the tricks rushing by, the excitement of men cruising for something I had. Just for that one moment, I got this high, like, see I can *still* do this, I can play the game; be in control. Do you know what I mean?"

I nodded, but I was speechless.

"This guy drove by in his Mercedes and well, I took care of him. Then, after he did a blast of coke, he started getting a little freaky on me. He told me if I was a whore, I wasn't even a good one and he pulled my head down and tried to make me go down on him a second time. His thing was making me gag; it had this terrible sour smell, and I felt like I was going to throw up all over his fancy Mercedes. Somehow, I managed to get out of his car. I heard him shouting at me that I was a dead woman the next time he saw me."

"Jesus," I said. "Maybe we should report him."

"Yeah right," Denise said. "And tell them one of San Diego's finest is a psycho john. No one would believe it."

"What do you mean San Diego's finest?"

"He said he was a high level cop. Anyway, after I got away I was so freaked out I almost used. I had an outfit in my hand and I broke the needle off of it."

"What's an outfit?" I asked.

"A syringe. One of the girls gave it to me. I was going to use chiva."

"What's chiva?"

"Chiva is what they call heroin on the streets."

I reached for her hand. "It must have been awful for you to get that close to your old ways. But the main thing is, you *didn't* use." Then I gave her a hug and I got all choked up again.

"Denise, you've been out there on the streets for years. You know there are guys like that cop all over the place. Don't you ever get scared out there?"

"When I hit the streets, I'm fearless," Denise responded without hesitation. "Another person takes over, and I let her run the show."

"Wasn't it weird being out there, I mean now that you know it's an addiction?"

"Yeah, it felt strange," Denise said, nodding. "Because I know that I don't have to be doing this anymore, and yet there I was again, one more time."

"What was it like on the boulevard?"

Late into the night Denise told me about what it had been like to go back out there. And then she told me about other nights, and other mornings, trapped in an endless twilight zone, a kind of hell, filled with shadows and dark, twisted desires. There in those shadows lurked men who were into cross-dressing, men with coffins in their rooms; men who wanted to be burned; men who wanted her to walk on their chests while she wore spiked heals, men who were into bestiality, violence, and complete degradation.

I felt a complex mixture of emotions—sadness, contempt for that world, and gratitude—gratitude that I hadn't ever gone down that far. Yet.

"Promise me," I said. "Promise me that you won't go back out there again."

"I promise. And you won't go to Kix, right?"

"Right," I said.

Denise spent the night on my couch. I guess you could say we were helping each other out. She was keeping me from going out and dancing and flirting and sometimes more at the neighborhood nightclub, and I guess I was keeping her from going out and turning tricks. *What a team!*

I hadn't talked about my past for all these years; that is, not until I told my little secret to a woman that I desperately wanted to look up to, a woman who I thought had risen above the sex industry. But Denise was still hooked into it, just as I was still hooked into the secret life, the forbidden and double life. That adrenaline rush I got from being bad.

I had wanted a role model. But Denise could not quite be cast in that role. She was treading on thin ice, about to fall in, and if I wasn't careful, I might just fall back in with her.

That night I had a hard time falling asleep. I felt completely confused. Was Denise in the life or not? Did she really want to change? Why did she want to go on national television, or even conduct interviews with local newspapers if she was still dabbling with the sex industry?

While Denise slept soundly on my couch, I paced. Patrick was out of town, on business. As I already mentioned, Patrick worked all week in Ventura County, and then commuted back to San Diego on the weekends. We were planning to keep it this way until I got married. But the truth was, I liked it this way. I was used to long distance relationships.

My relationship with my father was my original blueprint for long distance relationships. He had always lived 3,000 miles away from me. And when he was locked up, it felt as if he were on another planet.

Later that evening, when I finally did fall asleep, I had terrible nightmares. In the world of my dreams, I moved erratically through a dangerous maze. In one scene, I saw my stepfather chasing me. When he caught me, he molested me, and then gave me a necklace. "Don't tell," he warned me. "Or your mother might try and die again."

In the next scene of my dream, the man who, when I was fifteen, said he wanted to cut my breasts off and take them with him, chased me down an endless road. No matter how hard I tried, I couldn't find my way out of the maze.

I woke up bathed in sweat. I rubbed my eyes; the dream world darted in and out; a series of disjointed images, a snapshot of my fragmented, wounded psyche. It didn't take me long to figure out what the dreams represented. I hadn't healed from my experiences as a prostituted woman. My new friendship with Denise was giving me a chance to look at my past. And although my compulsions to act out were on a different scale than Denise's, I was still split between two disparate worlds.

One of my worlds seemed normal enough, at least on the outside. I was a professional woman. I was engaged to be married. It was to be a big Catholic wedding in an elegant, archdiocese approved church.

But my other world was hidden. A sexual underground. The dark side. My shadow side. My journey, my quest, was to integrate, embrace and accept this dark side. Only then would I be truly whole.

When I woke up Denise was gone. The phone rang twenty minutes later.

"Hey—where'd you go?" I said.

"I went home. Look, there's a reporter from the San Diego Sun who wants our story."

"For what?"

"I called the paper and told them we were starting a Sex Industry Survivors Meeting at the YMCA," Denise said.

I just listened.

"She wants to interview us tomorrow. Can you do it?"

"Yes," I said. "I think I will."

chapter sixteen

We agreed to meet in the lobby of the San Diego Sun. Our illustrious group included Denise, Joanne, the notorious former high-tech madam and founder of Sex Industry Survivors Anonymous, and me of course.

A reporter rushed toward us. She was a crisply dressed young woman, an intern in her early twenties. "Thanks for coming out," she said, leading us into a conference room. "I'm Jennifer."

Denise introduced us. "This is Joanne, the Founder of Sex Industry Survivors Anonymous." Then, she introduced me. "And this is Cathy." We had agreed before the meeting that I would use a fake name.

We all sat down at a large table and Jennifer handed us each our own bottle of water. "So, how did you guys get into this?" she said, looking right at me.

I paused for a moment, struck with how odd it felt to be on *this* side of the interview process. For many years I had moonlighted as a freelance reporter for various San Diego magazines and newspapers. For a while, I even had my own column in a small alternative newspaper. I wondered how the editors of these publications would respond to my writing if they knew about my previous line of work.

My stomach all tied up in knots, I finally replied. "I needed money to pay my college tuition."

"You earned money for college through…that is—"

"Through prostitution," I said, finishing Jennifer's sentence. "I wasn't able to pay for my tuition by cleaning houses or working at Friendly's ice cream parlor. A lot of that had to do with the fact that I was drinking and using drugs. I really couldn't function at normal jobs. My friend told me about a job where I could earn all the money I wanted, and still do the drugs."

"And do you think that prostitution is an addiction?" Jennifer asked.

"Yes, I'm beginning to see that it is," I said. "Toward the end of my prostitution days I was obsessed with getting as many sugar daddies as I could. One guy wasn't enough; I had to have as many guys as I could get."

"What about you Denise—how did you get into it?"

"I started into prostitution when I was 18," Denise said. "I was a virgin. I had never had sex before. I turned my first trick in a cemetery. A guy gave me twenty bucks and I gave him a blowjob behind a gravestone."

"Do you remember how you felt after that?"

"I felt dirty and humiliated. But it was better than being at home."

The reporter continued scribbling notes. "And so you're the founder of this group?" she stated matter-of-factly, looking right at Joanne.

"Yes," Joanne said. "I started this group because there wasn't any other group like it."

"When I did my research," Jennifer said, consulting her notes, "I heard you were called the High-Tech Madame. You were formally known as Rene Ravel. You were grossing $30,000 a month from the operation, which was equipped with closed-circuit television to screen arriving customers and a VCR that played porn videos 24-7. You spent three months in jail, and your mother served a one month sentence."

"Yes," Joanne said. "Your research is correct—that's how it went. It was my time in jail that made me start to look at what was happening to me. And I saw that there were a lot of misconceptions about prostitution."

"Such as?" asked Jennifer.

"There are some misunderstandings that prostitution has to do with sex addiction but it doesn't. Some of our members don't even have sex with their clients. Some people think they have problems with drugs. Over one-third of our members never even touched drugs. We feel that what we have is an addiction to the sex industry itself."

The reporter looked in Denise's direction. "Do you feel that's what you have—an addiction to the sex industry?"

Denise nodded vehemently. "One of the reasons that I was out there was that I loved the excitement. I also loved the power and control I thought I had. I now realize that every trick I ever turned was my way of taking revenge against my father because he was so abusive."

"I'm sure that just having a place where you can go to tell the truth is very beneficial," Jennifer said, in a strangely upbeat tone.

I nodded. "I just went to my first meeting last week. Before that meeting I hadn't ever talked about my involvement in the sex industry."

"Many women have never been able to tell the truth about their involvement with the sex industry," Joanne commented. "It's a tremendous fear that many members have. In fact, some women have been carrying fears of their husbands finding out to the point that they have constant nightmares, or anxiety attacks."

"I feel so much shame about my past," I blurted out. "Other than my sister, no one knows what I've been through. I never told my former husband, and I still haven't told my fiancé."

"What do you think your fiancé's reaction might be?" Jennifer enquired.

I glanced down. "It scares me too much to even think about that."

Jennifer directed her next question to Joanne. "How did you structure the group?"

"We based it on the 12 steps of recovery formulated by Alcoholics Anonymous," Joanne stated. "We wanted to provide refuge for former male and female prostitutes, pimps, madams, and former porn actors who've had sex for money."

"How do you get people help for this addiction?" Jennifer asked.

"We give them a place to start talking about what happened in their past, or for some, what's happening in their present." Joanne said. "Many individuals want to get out, but have no way to go about it. They think it's their only means of support. Often, they don't even consider that whatever aspect of the industry they are into really counts as sex work. You'll hear stuff like, 'Oh well he never touched me,' or 'I'm an exotic dancer—that's not prostitution.' Talking honestly about what's going on not only helps break through denial, but also takes the power away from the addiction and empowers the individual."

The reporter looked puzzled. "If women can get addicted to the sex industry, what elements fuel that addiction?"

"When people are addicted to the sex industry, they crave attention, money, and power," Joanne answered.

"Was that the experience you had, Denise?"

"I was definitely into the money, and the control," Denise told Joanne. "I thought I had power over the john, because I could tell him what was going to happen, how long it was going to take and how much it was going to cost. It's still hard for me to look at myself in the victim role because while I was in the industry, I felt like it worked for me. I loved the money. I hated the sex."

"How about you Cathy, did you feel like you were in control?"

Tears welled up in my eyes. "I tried to be in control, but I never really felt like I was. No matter how hard I tried to control the game, it always controlled me. Sometimes I think of myself as a 'failed hooker.' I started off working for a madam and then I tried to steal her clients and turn them into sugar daddies."

No one said anything for a moment, and the silence was making me nervous. I sighed with relief when Joanne finally spoke up. "Getting out of the life is tough. Not only is there the emotional aftermath and sexual problems to deal with, but just adjusting to the mundane can be tough."

"What do you mean by that?" the intern prodded.

"Some prostitutes miss being told how sexy they are, or the constant excitement. Everything changes, like you can't stay up all night. A lot of us had people cleaning our houses for us. We have to learn how to do things like that. Usually it takes about two years to settle down and get into the swing of things."

"What are some of the difficulties you've had in reaching out to women who want help?" Jennifer asked.

"Most are very isolated. They don't read newspapers, magazines, or talk to each other. They *do* watch TV. I've started a major media campaign. So far I've had four appearances on *Geraldo*, and two on *Sally Jesse Raphael*.

"Are law enforcement officers helpful?"

Joanne nodded. "Now they are—since they know I'm legit. In our first year, they kept trying to bust me. They thought it was just a game. They even sent an undercover cop to my work pretending to be a telephone repair-man."

"Do you think that our story will be on the front page?" Denise said.

Joanne and I exchanged glances.

"I really couldn't tell you that," the reporter said. "If I can get it to run on the front page, is that something you'd like?"

"Yeah," Denise admitted, "I always wanted a story about me to run on the front page of a newspaper."

I just nodded, once again quietly struck by the irony of the situation. As a struggling freelance journalist, of course I too had wanted to place a front-page story. But *not* a story that was about me—especially a story about my checkered past.

chapter seventeen

After the interview, we all went to a small deli on the bottom floor of the building and ordered lunch. We then carried our sandwiches, just like the secretaries and other professionals, into a small, concrete courtyard.

I noticed that beads of sweat were collecting on Joanne's forehead. "I thought it went really well—what did you two think?" she said.

For some reason, I had the insane urge to laugh.

"Are you okay?" Joanne said.

"Yeah," I said, biting into my sandwich. But I wasn't okay. Frankly, it broke my heart to talk about my life as a failed hooker. My only hope was that perhaps someone might read the article and think twice before entering into prostitution.

As I continued to study Denise I noticed that nothing seemed to get to her. "It doesn't bother you one bit, does it?"

"What doesn't bother me?"

"Talking about the past."

She just shook her head. Frankly, I thought there was something strange about her lack of emotions.

"So, how are your wedding plans coming along, Juliet?" Joanne asked.

"My wedding plans?"

"You are getting married, aren't you?"

"Yes."

"Do you plan on telling him about your past?" Joanne persisted.

"Of course I do," I said indignantly.

"When?"

I felt my blood begin to boil. I would tell him when I was ready to. I wanted to get married and yet I wasn't sure Patrick would want to marry me if I told him. How do you explain something like that to someone like him?

"Look, the reason I want to know is that I want you girls to come with me on the Donahue show," Joanne explained.

"The Donahue show—" I said, feeling my heart race.

"I want to do it, that's for sure," Denise bubbled.

"But aren't you afraid people will recognize you?" I said.

Denise and Joanne looked back and forth between each other. "We want people to recognize us," Joanne said. "We want to set an example for other women. We want to show them that there's another way to live."

"Well, I'm not going on the Donahue show," I replied emphatically. "Or any show."

No one said anything. Finally, Joanne told us she had to get back to L.A. "I don't want to get stuck in traffic."

We watched her walk away. I bit into my roast beef sandwich and watched the office workers in the courtyard. But I wasn't even really seeing them, and I wasn't even really tasting my food.

* * *

1976
San Francisco

I was seventeen. Seventeen and just about homeless. My father had kicked me out one more time. I had been on job interview after job interview and I just wasn't qualified to work in an office. No one wanted to hire me.

I was terrified. That same morning, a man who was most likely a pimp propositioned me. "Hey little girl," he said. "Can I buy you a cup of coffee?"

I didn't answer him; I continued walking. He followed close behind. "What makes a girl like you so aloof?" he asked.

"Just leave me alone," I snapped.

"Bitch," he muttered under his breath. "I'll meet up with you next week and you'll beg me to talk to you."

A thousand unseen eyes leered at me. A cacophony of male voices hooted at me, howling at me like dogs. Tall skyscrapers were closing in on me. I started to split off from myself. From this perspective, the horror I felt subsided.

* * *

"Juliet—Juliet, I'm talking to you," Joanne said.

"What?"

"You dripped mustard on your shirt."

"Oh," I said, peering down at my once pristine white shirt. Sure enough, a large circle of mustard now decorated my blouse. I rushed into the nearest restroom for damage control.

I felt stained by my past and stained by my present. And no matter how much I tried, I knew that the stain, like the memories of my painful past, might never come clean. I crawled into the restroom stall and I began to sob.

"I'm going to go on the Donahue show," Denise said. "I don't understand why you don't want to."

"I don't even have the nerve to tell my fiancé and you want me to go on the Donahue show?"

Denise and I were standing near a traffic light in downtown San Diego. Joanne had returned to Los Angeles. A rail-thin black woman strode past. It looked like a clump of her matted black hair was about to fall out, as well as what was left of her soul.

"Sometimes when I walk down the street I know people think that I'm a ho'," Denise said. "Do you ever feel that way?"

"I was never on the streets."

"Oh that's right, you was a high-priced call girl. Well, you go girl," Denise said, breaking into her perfect black girl accent.

I laughed, feeling suddenly lighthearted. When I was with Denise I think I reverted back to being about seventeen years old. The light changed, and when we went to the other side of the street, Denise said, "I've been thinking about dancing again."

I stopped dead in my tracks. "Here we go again. You want to go on national television and talk about being a recovering prostitute when you're still in the life."

"I said I was thinking about it," Denise snapped back at me.

A group of Japanese tourists complete with cameras strode past. Denise waved at them. They snapped pictures, excited.

"But you told me you called an escort service—that you did an in-call."

And then something registered. Denise's indifference, her lack of emotions. There was a reason for it. She was still a player. "We need to talk," I said.

I took her by the elbow and dragged her into a coffee house. It was one of those artsy places with fuchsia and ochre walls and artworks that were surreal and amateurish. I had always liked this place—it was right at the corner of J Street and Island, or crackland U.S.A.

As I sat there with Denise at the corner table shaped like a fish I watched the traffic going in both directions. The huge windows gave me the feeling that I was literally right there, in the heart of the city, with the swoosh of the cars going past on either side, as I watched crack-addicted prostitutes hit on middle-aged johns in Lincoln Continentals.

Normally, when I sat here, I felt a sense of exhilaration, a feeling that I was one of the lucky ones—I had risen above this tawdry world. But today I didn't feel that sense of separation from the sex industry. I didn't feel like just an observer, and all the property lines that I imagined between my past and my present seemed blurred, if not non-existent.

Now I just felt exposed, and the cars going past on either side made me nervous. I looked down at the fish eyes embedded in the table; one of them seemed to have winked at me.

"Are you out of the business or not?" I said to Denise, after they brought us our coffee.

"You think it's that simple, don't you?"

"Isn't it?" I demanded. "It's either you're in it, or you're not."

"Is that right?" Denise shot back. "I guess you think because you have a good job in the computer industry, and you're getting married that you aren't in it anymore."

"But I've been out of it for ten years," I insisted.

"You might have been out of the life, but believe me, the life's still inside of you. It's going to take you a few more minutes to get yourself back together again."

"I've been clean and sober for—"

"Yeah, but you're not clean on the inside," Denise said vehemently. "Spiritually, you a ho' still, just like me."

"How can you say something like that?"

"You keep trying to pretend the whore in you never existed.

Believe me, until you embrace the ho' in you, you'll never be free."

"I have no idea what you're trying to say," I said.

"I'm talking about being free," she said. "I'm talking about being free from the inside out. I'm talking about being able to tell the truth—especially to yourself."

"I still have no idea what you're getting at."

"You can take the girl off the streets but you can't take the street out of the girl, that's what I'm getting at."

Exasperated, I shook my head.

"You're having affair after affair because you know damn well your engagement and upcoming marriage is a big fat lie," Denise went on, relentless. "You try to tell yourself that after you're married you'll start over, wipe the slate clean, and forget everything you've been or done. But you're branded, Juliet. You're one of us."

"No, I'm not. Not anymore. I'm out of here," I said, and tried to get up, but she grabbed my wrist.

"No," Denise countered. "I'm not letting you run away. You've been doing that all your life."

I looked at her, scowling.

"You can't just ride off into the suburban sunset and become little Miss middle class happily married girl," Denise went on.

"Why not?" I persisted. "Why can't I? Why are we giving our stories to reporters and starting up Sex Industry Survivor's groups then?"

She flipped her hair back and peered into the hard red eyes of the fish-shaped coffee table. The eyes embedded into the coffee table were made of abalone shells.

"I guess it helps to talk about it, but I'm not sure I'm really ready to stop," she explained candidly. "Sometimes the urge just hits me. I think about earning five hundred dollars. That's the magic number; the big five. By the way, I know this guy who wants to meet you. He wants a threesome."

"A threesome? What the hell are you talking about? You aren't actually…no, I don't believe you—did you mean what you just said?" I shook my head, dumbfounded. "I'm getting really confused here."

"I was just telling you what's inside my head, I wasn't telling you I was planning on doing it."

"Don't you think we have to choose, Denise?"

"Oh, it's like that is it," she snarled. "Well, then, what about you?"

"What do you mean what about me?" I said.

"Have you really made the choice to be out of it, completely?"

"Of course I have."

"Well then what about that guy who promised you a gold bracelet if he could watch you and another girl?

"What about it?"

"That's prostitution, Juliet."

"That's ridiculous," I said, but then my gut tightened, and I had this bad feeling that maybe she was right.

"It's an exchange. A sexual fantasy in exchange for a material item. What, do you think the only way it counts as prostitution is when cold, hard cash is involved? We work our game all kind of ways. Don't we?" she persisted, her blue eyes narrowing into slits.

I almost felt I was getting hypnotized by the way she was looking at me. Then, she did something that really threw me off. "Don't we," she repeated, rubbing my hand up and down.

I just stared at her hand for a moment and this vision of my stepfather doing the very same thing to me as a young girl flashed through my mind. He would come into my room, and rub my hand, then move up my arm, and just keep moving up and down, really suggestively.

"I really don't know what you're talking about," I said finally, and then I yanked my hand away.

We both sat there in silence, and I watched the traffic going one way down Island, and then, after the light changed, in the other direction, down J street. Another scrawny crack ho' disappeared into the temporary luxury of a trick's shiny ride. I grimaced, remembering. Despite the effects of the double latte, long buried pain had erupted.

All the truths and stories I had told myself about my past now seemed questionable. All of a sudden I wasn't sure who I was. My involvement in the sex industry had warped my ability to see the truth about myself. I had an entirely different set of values and belief systems. And even though I had been sober a while, I didn't have a fully developed conscience.

Because I first got involved with the sex industry in my late teens, I was robbed of that chance to build an appropriate bridge to adulthood. I would have to begin to build a new foundation. I would have to start over. I guess I thought that quitting drinking would be enough. But that was only the beginning.

My journey had just begun.

chapter eighteen

August 1991
Downtown San Diego

A large woman in a flowery print dress handed us a flyer as we entered the nearly empty art gallery. She gestured towards the photographs that lined the walls. "These are the pictures of the 45 women who have been brutally murdered in San Diego County in the last three years."

Denise walked up to one of the photographs. "I knew this girl. She was the one who squealed on that cop. I heard they found her with rocks stuffed in her mouth."

I moved closer to the picture to get a better look. "How horrible."

Undaunted by our discussion, the art gallery representative continued on with her description of the exhibit. "All these women were thought to be NHI—which is a police term that stands for No Humans Involved, meaning that the victim's lives were not considered to be important. Transients and drug addicts get the same status."

"So, let me get this right," I said. "Are you saying that if the police think that the victim was a prostitute they aren't even considered human?"

She nodded. "But not all of these women were prostitutes," she explained, leading us to another picture. "This woman, for example, was an office clerk. She had a husband and two little girls. When her car broke down, she just happened to be in the wrong place at the wrong time."

The woman in the black and white photograph looked familiar to me. As I stood there looking at her image time stopped.

"Did you know her?" Denise asked.

"Yes, I mean no," I stammered. "I didn't know her—but in a way, I did."

"What do you mean?"

I stood in the center of the room. I turned and I looked at each face. "These were all my sisters," I explained. As I looked at each picture, I realized that each face represented a woman who had been someone's mother, wife, sister, daughter, or even someone's best friend. Each woman had once been part of a family, a church, and a community. Each face on the wall represented a woman's story that would never be completed because now she was dead.

A chill went through my very being as I realized a stark, cold fact. My face could have been up there on the wall. *Framed. Matted. Just another Jane Doe.*

I wondered, as I stood there in the gallery, why women perceived to be in the sex industry were scapegoated to such an extent that they wound up dead. I had read in a book about sexual deviance and crime that men who murder prostitutes often feel they are doing society a service. They believe that they are ridding the streets of evil women. It is also true that in times of war, the enemy is always dehumanized. This dehumanization allows those in power to destroy their victims without remorse.

The sex industry is lethal on every level because it dehumanizes women. The sex industry turns women into objects for consumption and disposal.

I'm not even sure how long my friend and I stayed in the gallery. I felt that each woman had something to share with me, and so I stood in front of each photograph for a long time, listening, absorbing. Hundreds of years ago, these women might have been burned at the stake because they were thought to be witches. Now, instead, they were called prostitutes and murdered. As I looked from face to face I felt a potent anger brewing within me. But then my anger turned to pain and I started to cry.

* * *

I had just called my mother on the east coast. As I held the phone in my hand I was struck with the odd feeling that my mother was on another planet instead of 3,000 miles away. Since she didn't seem to have heard my last question, I tried again. "So, aren't you going to ask how the wedding plans are going?"

There was silence on the other end of the line, and then my mother finally managed to respond. "Your wedding plans. Oh yes. Well, of course. Did I tell you I'm taking piano lessons? I'm working on so many projects I really do not know where to start. My new medications are starting to work. The only problem is—"

"But mom, what about the wedding?" I interjected. "It's almost the end of August; the wedding is four months from now. Will you be there?"

"Yes, I will be, even though I think it's a mistake."

Maybe I was still upset about seeing all those women in the

gallery, but I was also getting upset with my mother. The little girl in me shrieked. One more time, my mother wasn't listening to me. One more time, what was important in my life was insignificant to her.

"*She's not ever going to be there for you,*" I heard the tough juvenile delinquent girl within me saying. "*Why don't you just give up? Your mother is an addict just like you. She's taken too many pills for too many decades. You know how it is. You grew up swallowing them like candy yourself. It doesn't matter. Doesn't matter if she comes to the wedding. Doesn't matter . . .*"

"I'm sorry you think my upcoming wedding is a mistake," I said softly, shifting back into my adult mode.

"It doesn't really matter what I think, does it? You're going to do what you want to do; you always do."

I chose to ignore my mother's sarcastic tone. "I went to an exhibit today," I said. "It was called 'NHI'." My mother didn't respond. "Mom, are you listening? Do you want to know what NHI means? It's a police term for 'No Humans Involved.' The media, along with the police, have implied that the forty-five women who have been murdered in San Diego County in the last few years were all NHI."

"Murdered—Niki, get down. That cat. Honestly."

"In the exhibit, they had pictures of all the murdered women."

"That's nice. God, I really wish this cat were a little less hyper."

"My picture could have been up there, Mom. I could have been one of those women."

"How can you say such a thing?" my mother asked. "Those women were probably all drug addicts and street prostitutes."

Like your daughter, I thought, but instead, I interjected, "They weren't all just that—some of them were mothers, or professionals. One of them was an insurance agent."

"Well, maybe they were living a wild lifestyle."

"Does that mean they deserved to die?"

"Oh Juliet, honestly."

"You don't seem to understand," I said, my voice becoming a shrill whisper. "What I'm trying to tell you is that could have been me. I was at a high risk."

"High risk? What are you talking about?"

"In a position to be exploited. I was young, pretty, and on my own when I shouldn't have been."

"Here we go again," my mother whined. "Am I ever going to stop hearing about what a poor mother I was?"

"I wasn't saying that you were a bad mother."

"Well then what *were* you saying? You just couldn't keep your pants on, that's all."

There was a long, pregnant pause while I took time to recover from the bomb my mother had just dropped. "Thanks, Mom, thanks a lot."

"I just get so tired of the drama, either it's you, or your sister, or—"

"I just wish I could have been a little more protected, that's all."

"How was I supposed to protect you when you were running away every five minutes?"

"If your husband would have kept his hands off me maybe I wouldn't have had to."

"Oh for God's sake," my mother shrieked. "I can't believe I still have to have conversations like this with my adult children."

"I just want to talk about my feelings."

"Well I don't. I don't want to talk about feelings. I'm sick to death of talking about feelings."

My mother was from that era that Betty Friedan wrote about in the book *The Feminine Mystique*. The book, published in the early seventies, launched the second wave of the women's movement. The book confronted the myth of the contented housewife. It turns out many women really weren't happy scrubbing their floors and raising children. They longed for a fuller life.

These women were given Valiums and told to conform. I inherited some of my mother's confusion about what it meant to be a woman. *Do not be too smart. Stand by your man. But have something to fall back on.*

Once, my mother told me a story from her teen days. A talented seamstress, she had won a dress-sewing contest. She was flown to New York City, where she was given a chance to model the dress on a runway.

"She could go so far, but she has no ambition," the judges said.

"I just didn't care about winning," my mother told me. "Girls weren't supposed to want to win, or have any kind of control or power over their destinies. When I was in my early twenties during the fifties, I believed that it was noble to be out of control."

It was easy to forgive my mother for not wanting to win, but how could I forgive her for not wanting to be a mother? When my stepfather wanted to have me committed because I wouldn't be sexual with him, I knew I was on my own, and so I ran away. I've been running ever since, trying to get back home.

At sixteen, I walked through the Haight-Ashbury, my only possession my father's ancient suitcase. Terrified and hungry, I knocked on the door of a person I had just met the day before. "Can I stay here for a day or two?" But the stranger, an older, middle-aged man, had plenty of other young teens keeping him company, and so I was turned away. Abandoned, scared and unprotected, of course I eventually became a whore. At least then I was in control.

All of it is churning inside of me now. My past. My present. My mother. My sister. Those women on the wall. The pain was overwhelming, and I could not shut it out. All I really wanted was for my mother to stroke my hair, to cradle me, and to tell me that she's sorry it had to go down the way it did; that she didn't really know how to mother me because she hadn't been mothered herself.

Or if she could just somehow tell me: *"Look how far you have come girl. You were in that life and you rose above it. But now, because you are not just an image framed on the wall, you can help other women choose a new life. You are a true survivor."*

But she isn't even on the phone anymore. She is playing a song on the piano for me. As I listened, I wondered if my mother would ever allow herself the opportunity of feeling her sadness instead of taking all those pills.

I told my mother I liked the song she was playing and I hung up the phone. I guess dealing with issues concerning my past right before my wedding wasn't the greatest idea. Besides, trying to talk to my mother about the past was *never* a good idea. After I hung up the phone, I remembered how when we were growing up, my mother had played the piano endlessly, her ubiquitous White Russian right there at her side. Sometimes, on the rare occasion that she would leave her drink unattended, I would help her finish it.

Out of nowhere, I felt like taking a drink. I didn't want to listen to, or feel, the pain of the wounded little girl within me. Didn't want to acknowledge that she had gone into hiding, and transformed herself into the defiant, destructive teenager.

In order to become whole, to become real, I would have to experience the pain of my disassociated self. To do that, I had to have the intention to learn about the pain of the little girl within. The pain then washed over me in waves. I grieved the loss of my innocence and I grieved the loss of my mother's unconditional love, and the forty-five dead women whose pictures were on the wall.

As part of my path in healing the good girl/bad girl myth, I needed to listen carefully to the painful cries of the wounded child within. This bonding with my inner child would heal the split between my false self and my real self.

chapter nineteen

September 1991
San Diego

I walked down to the newspaper stand at the end of our street to pick up the daily paper. Once I got home, I anxiously thumbed through the pages in search of the article that the fledgling reporter had composed about "Cathy," (AKA Juliet West) and the other founding members of Sex Industry Survivor's Anonymous. I was just beginning to read it when Patrick walked in.

"What's that?" he demanded.

"Oh, this?" I mumbled.

"Yeah, that," he snapped vehemently.

"It's nothing, really, just the Lifestyles section."

Patrick ripped the paper out of my hands. "Lemme see that—now."

I felt myself flinching as he read the headlines:

> ANONYMOUS GROUP OFFERS SEX INDUSTRY
> SURVIVORS REFUGE

"What the *hell* are you reading that for?"

"I'm a writer," I said. "I like to read well-written stories, that's all."

"Why do you have this fascination with the sex industry?"

"I don't have a fascination with the sex industry, it just happened to be in the paper, just like Anne Landers and the Astrology Section."

His face was starting to turn beet red, like it did sometimes, especially when he didn't feel I was measuring up somehow. I believe it had something to do with his Catholic upbringing, with being slapped around by nuns and all, but I can't be sure.

"You know something," he said, as he began ripping the paper into tiny pieces, "I'm beginning to wonder about you."

Patrick and I had decided to throw a small, impromptu pre-wedding dinner party. So far it wasn't going that well. I had invited Denise, and she appeared to be demonstrating some of the moves she had perfected while working as a stripper.

"I can't believe you invited her to our dinner party," Patrick snarled as he inclined his head in Denise's direction. "What could you possibly have in common with her?"

No acceptable response came immediately to mind, so I simply shrugged my shoulders.

"What'd she used to be, a stripper or something?"

"She's in recovery for all that."

"What the hell does that mean?"

I waited before I responded, especially since Patrick looked like he was practically frothing at the mouth. "She's trying to change."

"Yeah right," he said, vehemently tossing a bag of cashews into a too-small dish so that the crescent shaped nuts spilled onto the floor, ricocheting against the linoleum floor like tiny bullets.

I reached down to pick the cashews up. "It's an addiction," I explained.

"What's an addiction—stripping?" Patrick said.

Once again, I was speechless.

"I just don't understand how you could hang out with someone like that. She's nothing but white trailer trash."

Right at that moment Denise rejoined Patrick and I. "Thanks for inviting us," she said. "We don't get invited many places by people in AA."

I could tell Patrick was about to make a sarcastic retort, so I flashed him a "don't you dare say a word" expression.

"We're glad to have you," Patrick said. "What's a party without a little—"

"Color," I interjected. "Don't you love her outfit?"

"What there is of it is really nice," Patrick said, moving away from us and towards a circle of guests.

"Forgive him," I said.

"No wonder you don't want to tell him anything." Denise said. "He's very judgmental."

She was right. He was judgmental. That was why I was so afraid to tell him who I really was. Just then, I felt a pang of jealousy. I felt envious of Denise's marriage. Her husband knew she had appeared in porn. He knew she had been a stripper and a prostitute. He knew she had walked the streets 24 hours a day 7 days a week.

And yet he still accepted her.

"I got another call," Denise said. "We could make a lot of money."

"I don't get this," I whispered, glancing over my shoulder to make sure no one was listening. "You're here with your husband at a dinner party taking place in my house and you're asking me if I want to turn a trick?"

"Don't call it that, Juliet."

"What should I call it then?"

"It's an in-call; you go to the guy's house," Denise explained calmly. "You'd just be dancing for the guy. You wouldn't even have to touch him."

Again, I glanced around to make sure no one was listening. "Look, you can call it an in-call, or a date, or anything else to dress it up, but we both know what you're really talking about."

"What does all that have to do with what I asked you?"

I shook my head, exasperated. "If you don't know by now, then there's nothing I can say to explain it to you."

Rather than facing each other, we both glanced out at the guests in the living room. The guests, mostly friends from Alcoholics Anonymous, were eating chips with the onion dip I had just made for them. You know, the kind you make from Lipton's Onion Soup mix and sour cream. Patrick was telling the chip-eaters a story.

"Just this one last time," Denise pleaded.

"I thought we were trying to heal from being in the sex industry—not get back into it," I said forcefully.

She shrugged, and walked away. Just then, Patrick wrapped up his monologue and headed my way.

After the guests left, I invited Denise and her husband Cliff down to the jacuzzi for a soak. Patrick had already declined my offer. I guess the hot water made Denise feel like opening up and she started talking about how she had gone downtown last night and walked the streets by herself.

"I thought you said you were with Juliet last night," Cliff said.

"Well, I was for part of the evening, and then, oh okay, maybe I wasn't," Denise equivocated, immediately realizing she was busted. "I just felt like walking and I knew you would get worried about me."

Her husband looked at her like he was going to kill her. Then, without explanation, he got up, toweled off, and walked back towards my place. *Maybe he wasn't so accepting of her lifestyle after all,* I thought.

"What's up, Denise?" I asked. "What happened?"

"I guess I just love the night," Denise began to explain. "The nighttime is when I feel most alive. And then when a potential trick cruises by, I get this rush; it's almost like I'm euphoric. It's all about power. The power I know I have over him."

"You didn't have sex with anyone, did you?"

"You should see your face, Juliet. You look horrified. No; I didn't have sex with anyone."

"It's the first transaction that triggers the obsession," I said.

"There wasn't any transaction," Denise insisted.

"No, but aren't you playing with fire?"

"We both are."

That night, after all the guests had gone home, Patrick and I had sex. I lay there after he had fallen asleep, and I wondered if I really loved him. I wondered if I was even capable of real love after all I had been through. I knew I could never tell Patrick the truth. And I also knew that eventually the lies and secrets would divide us. But telling the truth—revealing my past—might do the very same thing.

I had several nightmares that evening. In one of them, I dreamt that someone had been murdered in my hotel room. I'm not sure who committed the murder. I believe the dream represents the blood of my past, spilling into my present. *In another recurring dream, a dark, demonic figure is chasing me and he wishes to do me harm. Who is he?*

I tried to not hang out with Denise much, as if, by distancing myself from her, I could distance myself from my own ambivalence. But then a series of events transpired that made me question whether or not the past really was the past. I met a young man who hinted that his family ranked among the 500 wealthiest families in the United States.

I started into old behavior—what I called the whorecon. This has to do with attempting to gain power through sex. Dressed as a Barbie Doll, I tried to con this young man into buying me lingerie and jewelry. I bragged that I possessed extraordinary sexual abilities.

So that he could test drive me, he brought me on board his private yacht. Much to my chagrin, my talents weren't exactly what I had made them out to be, and the young man never called me again after that night on his yacht.

What made me question my sanity was that even though the future millionaire clearly wasn't interested in me, I tried to contact him again. He ignored my calls. Feeling like a failed hooker one more time, I then became even more obsessed with having Tony buy me jewelry. Wasn't that a form of an exchange? Jewelry for sex. Sex for some sort of material compensation.

Was I really that different from Denise? Had I really recovered from the sex industry? I was about to walk down the aisle with a man I had little in common with. A man from whom I would have to deny my sexual past. Was I selling myself out one more time?

Denise says that to have secrets is to drink. Then I must still be drinking, since all weekend long all I could think about was Tony's promise of a gold bracelet, or how I might find yet another method to seduce that wealthy young man who owned the yacht. Feeling desperate, I looked through my old telephone and address book for someone, anyone to call. So far, there had always been willing participants and co-conspirators who would help to distract me from my own pain.

I felt insane—off kilter from the collision of two worlds. I could clearly see that I was still split into at least two very disparate selves.

There was the false self, the badgirl self, the partier, the temptress. Then there was the good girl about to be married in a Catholic church.

The split self, the false self ruled. I remember when I first felt her presence. It was during my mother's second suicide attempt. I was sitting by myself in the waiting room. I was fourteen. I began to disassociate; I began to split off from my authentic self. It didn't matter that my mother had just tried to die— at least that's what the split self told me. Suspended high above the waiting room, the split self began to sing.

Ever since our disastrous pre-wedding dinner party, Patrick and I had been fighting nonstop.

"You better not even think about inviting that whore to our wedding," Patrick snapped at me.

Without answering right away, I stared at my husband-to be. I was growing wearier by the minute. "What whore?" I whimpered, even though I knew exactly whom he meant.

"Denise—and I'm not going to get you a guard for your wedding ring until you produce a child."

"You can't mean that," I said, my voice a desolate whisper.

"You won't deserve it until then," Patrick stated emphatically. "And you'll need to get baptized. You need to be cleansed."

"I have to annul my first marriage and now you want me to get baptized too?" Patrick nodded. "What if I don't go through with it?"

"If you don't get baptized, I'll leave you here in San Diego, and you'll be forced to get a job—a real job. That'll put an end to all your so-called writing projects, won't it?"

I was between jobs as a technical writer, mostly because after many years behind a desk, I was experiencing neck and back challenges. One morning, I simply couldn't get up out of bed. I was placed on disability and sent to a physical therapist three times a week. At this particular moment in time I had been on disability for six months. Sure, it was true that I was using this recuperation time to catch up on my novel writing, but it's not like this was a crime or anything.

And I wasn't ready to go back to the "real" world, and so I agreed to get baptized. "Okay," I said to my husband-to-be. "I'll get baptized and I'll annul my first marriage."

"Good girl," Patrick said.

"Were you always pure?" the Catholic priest asked.

"Yes," I responded. "Pure and chaste."

"Sign here."

I did so. And of course my words were a lie. Rigorous honesty would cost me a diamond ring, a wedding, and the protection of a strong, white Catholic Irish male. It didn't matter that we had none of the same values. And it didn't matter that Patrick seemed quite displeased with the notion that his bride-to-be might be tainted with a checkered past.

Despite the many red flags, I was going to marry that man.

"You are now baptized, and your other marriage has been officially annulled," the priest said. "You may sign once more." He sprinkled water on us, blessed us, and after I signed the last document, sent us on our way. Ebullient, we walked out of the church.

I am going to be a perfect bride. I prepared for this big day by becoming a gift: a gift wrapped in satin and lace and expensive undergarments and something borrowed something blue something old something new and shoes dyed just the right color.

"Just climb into the dress," Denise said. "It's easier that way."

And so I climbed in, and just for that moment I was safely ensconced in dreamy folds of white. And then I lost myself in the perfection of the image I saw in the mirror. Everything about me that had not been pure melted away.

We are to be married at a Catholic Church called Immaculata, the Perfect Birth, which sits at the top of the hill in San Diego. Once I am veiled and about to be joined in holy matrimony to my more superior half I will be redeemed, and triumphant. No one will be able to question that I am now a good girl. The placement of my veil will indicate to all that I am protected, virginal, and untouched. I will walk towards the stained glass image of the Mother Mary, Queen of Peace, right behind Jesus.

Denise had accompanied me to the bridal store to try on dresses. For a moment, as she pulled the layers over my head, I felt trapped. An image I had seen in a *National Geographic* magazine flashed before my eyes. It was a picture of a woman wearing a burka, the traditional required wear for women in Afghanistan. It shrouded a woman from head to foot so none of that evil, tempting female flesh could lure unsuspecting males. The burka was more of a jail cell than anything else, and right now so was my prospective wedding dress.

"Where'd the hell did you go?" Denise complained. "I've been standing here holding your dress for twenty minutes practically."

"Undo the dress," I snapped.

"Whatever happened to please and thank you," Denise suggested.

"Get this thing off of me," I said. "I feel like I'm suffocating."

Once I was finally extricated from the mounds of fabric, I wondered how I would tell her what I had to say. I decided that it was now or never.

"You can't come to the wedding," I said to Denise, as she helped me out of the wedding dress.

"What do you mean I can't come to your wedding?" Denise said.

"Patrick said I can't invite you to the wedding."

"Then why am I here helping you choose a wedding dress?"

Dirty Garden

Dirty garden caught in the linen the dust the past
The war
Give us this day our daily bread
Mother feed us
If she could breathe she could be our savior
If she could stop mourning the loss she might act
It is over but she keeps slipping, falling
Holding herself back from being in full charge
One moment of dignity erupts in the young woman's breast
Choked hostility erupts like smog in a darkened womb
One moment of righteousness blown apart by
Where is that child
Where is that child?
The child doesn't belong to you, but still you must know.

If you are not Mother Nature
Then ride the umbilical cord out nowhere
Formless where is and what is the shape of your dignity
Before you do what you will you must do what you must
The Bible has you created in the likeness of man but not yet whole
There is no name for you as you stand in this dirty garden
Alone.

You are
A young woman soft without pride
Without child
Bleeding
A choice not to give birth, not now
Too young
Instead
She grows a destiny of her own.

Uprooted the young woman sits in the dirty garden
She is planting her own ideas like worlds being
Inseminated into bombs
She is centered by guilt
That guilt that sees dirt and knows there is light
There is light and breath.

She was never the daughter of Mother Nature
She was always bad, bad because she would not
Feed the rotting flowers in the dirty garden
Hungrily she continues planting her own ideas like worlds
Being inseminated into bombs
She will not use her love to destroy
She will never see herself again as an evil woman
She is just barely escaping tragedy as she stoops
To plant the seeds of her own dreams
She runs no longer from men's contempt.

Instead she stands separate
She is on her own
Each time she speaks she creates a universe
Each time she plants she creates herself whole
Fresh separate
Human.

chapter twenty

The compulsion to act out sexually set in that night as I lay there with my fiancé, staring up at the ceiling. He had climaxed via the traditional missionary position but I had not climaxed, since I required direct clitoral stimulation.

They've been trying to tell us for some time that women are supposed to climax via the missionary position, but anatomically, that isn't always possible. And yet many women have told me they feel embarrassed that they cannot climax through the missionary position. Despite my difficulties with regards to sexuality, there is one thing that I can claim. I know what makes me come, and I refuse to fake orgasms.

Anyway, my desire to act out wasn't just about not having achieved an orgasm. My desire to act out was about covering up anxiety and the nagging, gut feeling that I was forfeiting my real self so that I could package myself into an acceptable bride-to-be.

I was making a series of decisions that had little to do with my own values and beliefs. This was pretty typical for me, since I often wasn't sure what my values and beliefs were anyway. For example, I had signed official documents in the Catholic Church. I had agreed to be baptized, which I really did not want to do.

I had even annulled my first marriage, which I also did not want to do. I had not done any of these things because they fit the kind of person I believed myself to be. I did all of them to please Patrick. In addition I told Denise, who was pretty much my closest friend at the time, that she couldn't come to the wedding.

Unable to sleep, I went into the living room to work on my tapestry. Sometimes the needlework consoled me. But I kept looking at the back of the tapestry, where multi-colored strands of threads created a web of confusion. In comparison, the front looked pleasant, serene. A simple bouquet of flowers.

I was so focused on comparing the front of the tapestry with the back of the tapestry that I managed to jab myself with the sharp needle. "Ouch," I said, and stuck the bleeding finger in my mouth. Once more, I wondered when my inner, interior life, would match the exterior, outer life. And I wondered, when, or if, I would become whole.

Later that week, when Patrick had returned to Ventura to work, I was restless, moody and not comfortable in my own skin. Delving so deeply into the demons of my past made me nervous, and I needed a fix. I simply *had* to have sex. I found my prey the very next night at Kix, where I found most of my young men.

I wound up in a car with a stranger parked in a back alley behind a strip mall. Twenty minutes later, a patrolman shone his light in my car. His partner stood at his side, a disconcerting smirk playing on his clean-cut face.

"You all right?" the patrolman politely enquired.

"I'm just fine," I said, feeling my face turn a deep shade of red as I struggled to pull my pants up.

"What are you two doing parked back here?" His partner prodded.

"Well nothing—yet, that is, officer," my brilliant guest offered.

My heart was pounding dangerously fast.

"I want you two to get out of here—now," the other officer commanded.

Bad girl shame washed over me. What was wrong with me? Why did I need to act out in this way? I felt absolutely humiliated. That night, alone in my room, I shifted back into another time.

I am fourteen again. I'm running through the church. I sit down beside my stepfather and mother. My stepfather turns to my mother and whispers. "She's a bad girl. A tramp. She'll run away when she's sixteen."

* * *

I wondered, as I made my way through the Los Colinas Women's Jail, how much different I really was from the inmates. Had I really changed? Was I truly a reformed sex industry worker? Or was I still acting out old patterns, over and over again?

Only a thin line separated me from these women behind bars. I had a desire to change. To heal from my past. I had managed to stay sober and stop turning tricks, but something deep within me, something I couldn't quite name or grasp, still needed to be resolved.

"They're in there, waiting for you," sneered the guard, a member of the San Diego Sheriff's department. "Sex Industry Survivors—who came up with that name?"

I refused to dignify his question with a response.

"Suit yourself; don't answer me. Besides, it doesn't make any difference what the name is, believe me. Do you think any of these women are capable of changing? What a joke."

He looked me up and down, and it made my stomach queasy.

"Make sure you tell the ladies if they want to slip when they get out, to call me."

I just shook my head, disgusted. I was pretty sure there had to be some kind of rule against correctional officers talking that way about prisoners. But I wasn't naïve about the realities of the system, and I understood the mind-set of this guy. My father had certainly bent my ear on countless occasions about the abuse that went on between guards and prisoners. And in women's jails and prisons, it was even worse.

"By the way," the impertinent guard pressed. "What do you all *really* talk about?"

"They talk about what gentlemen you all are," I said, not bothering to minimize the sarcasm in my tone.

"I just bet," he said, snickering.

I showed the girls in Los Colinas Women's Jail the article about "NHI."

"According to this study, about 45 women have been murdered. By calling them prostitutes, their cases received almost no priority. And yet some of them were *not* prostitutes. How does that make you feel when you hear the term: No Humans Involved?" I asked.

"I know they don't think of us as human. We're the evil bitches. The prostitutes. They don't want to consider us human because they want to scapegoat us," Fantasy stated. "And besides, I think the police are involved. I've been out here for eight years and I've heard stories. I've heard it might even be the sheriff's department. You just know things like that out here."

"I think it's the same killer as the Green River Killer," an inmate named Stephanie interjected. "I think he moved here. I used to work the strip out in Seattle. I knew this trick from Seattle, and as soon as he moved to San Diego, the murders stopped there and started up here. One time he looked me up and wanted to date me. I knew that if I went out with him I might wind up dead—and it wasn't just cocaine delusions I suffered from."

"I think the cops are involved too," concurred a woman named Joelle. "This guy hit me with a wrench behind the head. I told him I would do anything he wanted me to. Then he told me he didn't care, that all he wanted to do was to bash my brains in. That's when I started to fight. Somehow I got away. I was in the hospital eight days. When I got out they said this other girl was found dead only a few yards away from where I had been. And for some reason the cops didn't want me to talk about what had happened."

"Yeah," Fantasy agreed. "Shit like that's happened to me. Cops acting strange, like they're trying to cover for each other. You know what it really is?"

"What?" I asked.

"They want the pussy for free," Fantasy said matter-of-factly. "So they set a trap for you. Pretty soon the cops own you just like the johns or the pimps."

Several of the women nodded.

"Anyway," Joelle went on, "Since the day I got beat up and the cops told me not to talk about it, I changed. I got hard, I guess." She started tapping her foot nervously. "Now, as soon as I get the money I try to take charge. It's dangerous out there today. There's a lot of men out there real angry at women, and they'll try and hurt you because some woman tried to hurt them. And believe you me, they don't care if you had nothing to do with it—they'll jack you in a second." She looked out the barred jail window. "But I'm sicker than the men are because the minute I get out of here I'll be right back on the stroll."

"What about you," I said, turning to a thin Puerto Rican woman with the name Rene tattooed on her wrist.

"I'm Treena and I could relate with what she was sayin' because I've had guys try to do bad stuff to me just to get back at other women. It really isn't safe out there anymore. I know it's my responsibility to change my ways." Tiny tears welled in the corners of her eyes. "I want out of the life so badly but I guess I'm addicted—addicted to using men."

"All you need is the willingness," I reassured the women.

"Is willingness gonna pay my rent?" Treena said candidly.

"I didn't say it was going to be easy," I said. "But it's worth it. Would anyone else like to share?"

"I'll share. My name's Tracey. All I know is that it's another person out there on the streets. I'm not sure who it is, but it isn't me. When I got here this homicide detective told me that I would be safe in here, cause this guy was stalking me. To tell you the truth, I'm afraid to get out of jail."

"There *is* a way out of jail," I insisted. "There's a way out of jail and a way out of the sex industry. You can change. I've been out of it for ten years. I've been working in the computer industry as a technical writer. Today, I'm a recovering prostitute."

"A recovering prostitute," one woman said. "Ain't that some shit. Once a ho' always a ho'."

Several Hispanic women in the back row shifted in their seats. They looked like they agreed with her. I was really beginning to wonder if my words had any impact at all. I was pretty sure that more than half of them were only here because it was slightly more interesting than reading old copies of *People* Magazine or watching reruns of *Cheers*.

But I kept throwing my recovery out there, like a fisherman threw out a baited hook, hoping that one day the truth of my words would gently pull at their hearts, and they would believe that change really was possible.

Maybe I shouldn't care so much, but I do.

"You know, it isn't like the movie *Pretty Woman* out there," I said. No one responded, and so I went on. "That movie was a big lie. Some of you have told me that you almost died out there. And that is the truth. There's a war against women out there."

"There ain't no war," said a black woman, who was primarily toothless, and weighed no more than one hundred pounds. "Just a lot of cracked out muthafuckas."

"Doesn't it seem like these guys consider prostitutes their enemy?" I said.

The dentally challenged woman shrugged.

I was swimming upstream—nothing I said seemed to make much of an impact. Still, I forged onward. "I quit drinking and I quit using drugs. I haven't been in the sex industry for over a decade. I found a higher power. I didn't have a belief in God and then my sponsor wrote the Lord's Prayer on a napkin. I came to believe," I said, "like it says in Step Two of Alcoholics Anonymous: Came to believe that a power greater than ourselves could restore us to sanity."

"Did you tell your fiancé about your past yet?" Fantasy wanted to know.

"Ugh, no I haven't," I admitted. "But I intend to."

"The good girlfriend intend to." Fantasy laughed good naturedly. "Ain't that some shit. You're in here talking about healing and how you're this new woman. Well then how come you can't tell your man?"

"He might not want to marry her if he finds out," Joelle said. "Isn't that it?"

I really couldn't argue with her.

I feel that coming here, to the jail, is one of the most positive things I do. It is grace in action. But for the grace of God, it could be me sitting in one of these plastic chairs, wearing jail attire; my dark roots growing out and my nails badly in need of a manicure. I just never got arrested, that's all. And so, in contrast, as a result of my sobriety, I get to sit in the front of the room wearing an amethyst colored blouse and a smartly-tailored skirt and share my experience, strength and hope.

But sometimes, even though I do receive many gifts from coming here, it is still very painful for me. It hurts to listen to these women. It hurts because I hear my story, and it reminds me of the "badgirl" role I tried to play out there. I forced the vulnerable little girl underground. And so now I have to acknowledge her presence, and believe me, it isn't easy. I know that underneath the inmate's jive jail talk is always that hurt little girl. And so I listen for her story, try to hear her language, her barely perceptible articulations.

When I move beyond the pain that comes naturally from identifying with these women, I became stronger. I integrate the dark aspects of myself that for years I had tried to deny.

And so as the women tell their stories I become whole. Because by hearing about their lives it reminds me of where I've come from and where I must never return to. With each story that I hear, I become lighter. I become free to reinvent myself.

"I wrote out my first step. I admitted I was powerless over the sex industry and my life had become unmanageable," the young woman said. "But I didn't feel anything."

"That will come in time. Remember, you were out there for many years and you had your feelings locked away. It will take time to heal," I assured the inmate. "And to change. All you have to do is be willing to do whatever it takes to change."

"I'm Lateshia."

"Hi Lateshia," I said cheerfully.

"I want to change, but like, when I get out, I be there in the hood, and it's the same ol' same ol'. Homies be clockin' you and expectin' you to fall, pimpin' your ass as soon as you get out of jail. And besides, you white, there's more for you to do."

"We all have different challenges, I guess, but as long as you have the desire, you can find a better life. You can get out of the sex industry," I said passionately. "If I can do it, so can you." There was a pause, and then I told the women it was time to end the meeting. "We'll close with the Lord's Prayer, but before we do, did I ever tell you—"

"Yeah," Fantasy interrupted. "How you wrote the Lord's Prayer on a napkin cause you never learned it growing up. Well I found Jesus since I been locked up."

"That's good. That's wonderful. I've just started to pray to my lady," I said.

"Who, the Virgin Mary? What are you, Catholic or something?" Treena said.

"No. I just wanted to put a female face on whoever I connected with."

Without touching hands, which was against jail policy, we formed a makeshift circle. Here, for just a brief moment in time, within this gray, dismal jail, something special took place. And then, we weren't in a jail anymore. We weren't behind bars. Through our prayers, we were lifted above Los Colinas, to a sacred, spiritual place.

We were women, daring to tell the truth about the sex industry. We prayed, and afterwards two women said if they were allowed to hug me that they would. Inch by inch they were letting me get closer to them. A small tiny part of that mysterious aspect of myself, that darkness I couldn't quite name or grasp, began to get lighter, and the hard indelicate shell around my heart began to slowly disintegrate.

Late

You a little fuckin' late
Mamma
I already done laid down wid' the man
Countless faces swarming over me
And now you say
Come home
But it's too late mamma
You say you want to rescue me
From the gutter
You called it
Hell the gutter is my home
By now

I wonder how things
Might have been different
If when he
Touched me
Down there
Or my sister
You didn't look the
Other way

Stood up
To the man
Said no
Not my daughter
Not my daughters
And now it's too late

I already been
Where I shouldn't a been
Crossed that line
Your little badgirl whore.

chapter twenty-one

Late September 1991
San Diego

Another typical Southern California day, warm and sunny. I had just had my hair bleached so blonde that it looked nearly platinum. As I turned my white 1988 Firebird Pontiac onto the Route 8 exit that would take me to Mission Valley in San Diego, I felt an adolescent surge of blonde power that came from just having my hair done and driving a muscle car.

My feeling of exhilaration was fleeting, however. I was headed to the pre-marital counselor's office. The fact that I, that is *we*, needed pre-marital counseling should have been an indication that maybe, just maybe, big trouble lay ahead.

"How did you feel about what we discussed in our last session?" Kathryn, the marriage counselor asked. I told her I wasn't sure how I felt. After considering her question for a moment, I decided to be honest. I told her about the affair I was having.

"Tony is a con and a liar. I think the reason that I keep buying into his lies is because I feel a desperate need to be loved." I hung my head. "I really want to stop having this affair. I really do."

"Yes," Kathryn sympathized. "I'm sure you do."

"I told him that even though I am engaged, I still expect to be treated with respect. I told him that his words and actions have been hurting me. I let him hear my true feelings and emotions."

"That's good. We have to let people know when they hurt us. That's one way to protect your inner child. Keep picturing the little girl within you and know that you are protecting her and that you love her and that you will always be there for her."

I nodded and smoothed out my almost platinum blonde hair.

"Why don't you talk to the little girl inside of you right now," she suggested.

I tried to talk to my little girl inside but she didn't want to come out.

"It's your first time, isn't it?" she said.

I wanted to tell her that no, this wasn't the first time I had met my inner child but that she was probably hiding right now. Instead, I said, "The badgirl juvenile delinquent teenager within me is running the show right now."

"That's a perceptive insight."

She was right, it was perceptive of me, but just bringing that up hurt like hell, and my throat started feeling very tight, as it often did when the pain I should have experienced years ago would mix together with what I couldn't really experience now either. And so in order not to feel what I was starting to feel, I changed the subject. "I want to quit having affairs," I claimed. "But at the same time I keep feeling the urge to have just one more fling before I walk down the aisle. Do you mind if I pace?"

The therapist smiled at me for a moment and said, "Pace away."

"I must sound absolutely ridiculous. One more fling before the alter. One more night of passion. Which leads to...desperation and guilt and obsession and cut fingers...see this finger?"

I held up my bandaged pinky finger. "Cut it when I was busy planning my next tryst with man A, B, or C. My fiancé came up behind me and I guess I felt so guilty over what I was thinking about that I cut myself while slicing tomatoes for the tacos."

She nodded in the direction of my pinky finger. "That must have been very painful."

"Yeah it was," I acknowledged. "You know, maybe I keep having these affairs because I'm afraid of marriage." I walked over to her desk and picked up a picture of Kathryn in her younger days with a man I assumed was her husband. "How long have you been married?"

"Fifteen years," Kathryn replied.

"Fifteen years?" I repeated, stunned by the longevity.

Kathryn laughed. "Does it seem inconceivable?"

"Yes, I mean, no, that is, well, maybe it does," I was forced to admit. "I guess I've always associated marriage with death."

"That certainly is an interesting...association."

"I watched my mother's marriage from the age of three until I was legally an adult. She was miserable. She kept making suicide attempts. Maybe that's when I learned to associate marriage with death. The first time I was married, in 1982, I was only 22. I cried on my wedding night. I told my husband that I felt like a part of me was dying. He didn't look too happy about that."

"You look sad, Juliet."

So that I might attempt to feel my feelings for a change, instead of running from them as I normally did, I decided to sit back down. "I just wish I could talk to my mother, but whenever I try to talk about anything real, she shuts me out."

"Can you give an example?"

"Yeah, I can give a major example," I said. "I saw this art exhibit where they showed photographs of 45 women that had been murdered. I told my mother that I could have been one of those women—my photograph framed and matted and hanging on the gallery wall. But my mother didn't want to hear it. She always tells my sister and I that we're both too emotional. What's wrong with being emotional?"

"All you want her to do is listen, isn't it?"

"Yeah. I just want her to acknowledge all the times she dumped me off with strangers. My father did that too. But she doesn't want to hear about any of it! And what makes me feel the saddest is the fact that my mother didn't know what I was doing. How could she have been so blind? Did she think men just gave me designer clothing because I was sweet? The only time she ever came to get me was when she finally summoned up the courage to leave my stepfather for good. But by then it was too late."

"What was too late?" she asked.

"By then, I was already turning tricks in order to earn my way through college."

"Does Patrick know about your past?"

"Why does everyone keep asking that? I mean it's not like you can't rise above it. Anyway, you know what my mother said? She said she thinks I'm trying too hard to fit a square peg in a round hole. Meaning in other words, Patrick and I have nothing in common."

"And what do you think?"

"Oh, we'll work it out. I just believe that no matter what, love conquers all. That's why I chose 'Ain't no Mountain High Enough' for the first song to be played at our wedding."

"And what does that particular song mean to you?"

"It means, quite simply, that there ain't no mountain high enough to keep me from marrying this man. Not alcoholism, incest, drug and alcohol abuse, fear of commitment, fear of authority or fear of organized religion."

"I see, well your optimism is a good sign," she said, and then placed her fingertips together and peered at me. "When we first started talking you mentioned that you wanted to quit having affairs. Perhaps you have affairs so that you can be in control. Or, marriage might represent another form of prostitution to you. So if you have affairs, you're still calling the shots."

Thinking about what she said, I slouched back in the chair, linking my arms behind my head. "So, it's a control thing, is that what you're saying?"

"Perhaps," Kathryn replied cautiously.

"Or maybe I'm just trying to have all the sex my mother never had. Sometimes I feel that I'm addicted to the power I have over men."

"Or you might use sex to create distance," she ventured.

"Your guess is good as mine," I said, shrugging. "All I know is that I've been going into a jail dressed in a business suit telling other women that they can get out of the life."

"You should feel proud of your efforts to help those women."

"I do feel proud," I admitted. "But I also feel phony sometimes."

"Phony, and how is that?" Kathryn probed.

"I tell the inmates that they can change, that they can get beyond their mistakes. But have I?"

"You're sober, you're college educated, and you have supported yourself for many years as a technical writer. You're a professional woman, Juliet."

I nodded. "I know you're right, but while you were saying those nice things about me, I couldn't really hear it; it was like you were talking about somebody else. I don't know why it's so hard for me to hear nice things about myself."

"We'll work on that. We'll start by me affirming you again, and I want you to simply say thank you after I'm done. Ready?"

I nodded. "Fine. In addition to being a professional woman,

you have also worked very hard to continually develop your creative writing abilities. You just completed a certificate in writing at a local university that you told me took five years of night classes. Going to school at night like that takes an incredible amount of persistence."

"Thank you," I managed, although the words seemed unnatural.

"Well, you deserve the compliments. You never give up on your dream to be a writer. All that takes courage."

"Thank you, really."

"You see, Juliet, you're a contributing member of society, whereas incarcerated women are usually not."

"That's not what I really meant though."

"What then?"

"I mean that I understand the thrill women in the sex industry get from maintaining that illusion of control over a man. We all have a dark side. A dark side that we're all afraid to look at. Right now, I'm still ruled by that dark side. Maybe I am a bad girl after all. Where does being good get you? Do you know all along, my mother also wanted to be a writer? Yes. She did. She was, she is, so talented."

"I'm not sure how what you are telling me is connected, are you?" she said softly, attempting to be patient with me.

I thought about what Kathryn was implying, but how could you explain beliefs, motives and attitudes so deep-seated that they had colored your life for decades? Maybe I was trying to say that I felt my mother had sold out both her dreams, and her children. That she seemed like the ultimate victim and so I had decided to be nothing like her. Whatever long-buried truth I was digging for, I better unearth it and discuss it, and fast, because Kathryn was glancing at her watch.

"I guess what I'm getting at is that my mother was terrified of her talents. At one time, she wanted, like me, to be a writer. But she gave up on all that because when she was about 19 or 20, which would have been 1954, she believed that it was *'noble for a woman to be out of control.'* In other words, the more passive, out of control you were, the more of a woman you were. So she let's her crazy husband, my stepfather, terrorize an entire household for seventeen years."

"Thinking about all that really stirs things up for you, doesn't it?"

"I don't know, yeah sure, I guess. I mean of course it does."

"Stay with your emotion right now, Juliet. What is it you feel?"

"I just get mad, or maybe it's not mad, but frustrated, at my mother. Why couldn't she have been stronger? Why couldn't she have fought for what she wanted out of life? Or at least fight for us, fight for her children."

"As you've mentioned, in your mother's generation, women didn't have the freedoms they enjoy today. Sometimes we have to remember that we are victims of victims." Kathryn paused for a moment. "Perhaps you rejected any identification with your mother because you saw her as a victim. You saw that the sex addict in the family, your stepfather, had all the power. And so you came to the childish conclusion that power was attained through sexuality. This conclusion, or belief, created a blueprint."

"So how do I change the blueprint?" I asked.

"We keep chipping away at your beliefs," Kathryn replied. "It's like going on an excavation."

I nodded, just taking it all in.

"What is it, Juliet? What hurts now?"

"I guess I haven't forgiven her for looking the other way for all those years, and then when I had already been out there, she comes to 'get me out of the gutter.' It was a little late."

She thought for a moment and asked, "What story do you play over and over?"

"What do you mean?"

"Think about it. Aren't there stories, or scenes, little mini-movies that you play over and over in your mind? Tell me one of your stories again, and it will lose the power it has over you."

I sat back in my seat. I felt like I was falling. I closed my eyes.

*　*　*

1980
Baltimore, Maryland

My mother stood before me. She was not in good shape. I could tell she'd been drinking. "What brings you here today, mother?"

"I'm leaving him," she said. "I'm finally leaving your stepfather. And I've come here to get you out of the gutter."

Get me out of the gutter, I thought. *But it's my home—why bother?* After all, I had already been involved with drugs, sex and prostitution for several years now.

My mother looked around my current residence. She picked up a framed photograph of a young woman wearing a cap and gown. "Who is this person?"

"She's a law student, away for the summer. This is her room and she'll be back any day now."

"You mean you can't stay here?"

I shook my head. "I'm used to that kind of thing, Mom."

"How long can you go on living this way?"

"Living what way?"

"From place to place, man to man," my mother said.

"How nice of you to be so concerned," I shot back.

My mother placed the photograph back on the dresser where she had found it. She turned towards me and said, "My friend's daughter was murdered."

"Murdered?"

"Yes. They found the body last week. I went to the funeral with my friend. She is devastated. Her daughter was the same age as you."

I said nothing.

"I refuse to let that happen to my daughter."

I'd already been on the streets for four years. I had been a player in the sex industry all that time. Who knows how many times I had escaped death? I frowned and stared at my mother's purse, wondering how much money she might happen to have in it.

"I want you to come back home and live with me and your little brother. I'm getting an apartment. I'm finally leaving your stepfather."

In all my years out there, I had begged to come home. If my stepfather didn't want me for his own sexual purposes, then I couldn't come home. Or, if he couldn't control me in other ways, I was asked to leave.

And now she was finally leaving him, and she said she wanted to rescue me. Well, it was more than a little late, but I didn't say anything. Instead, I just looked at her purse on the table. It was wide open, and I could see a package of cigarettes, and her wallet. Normally my mother didn't smoke, but I guess she was drinking and smoking to get through what she was trying to do. I knew all about that. By the time I was 15, I was already a full-blown alcoholic and addict.

"I'm glad you're leaving John, but I'm fine where I am, and besides, Mom, I really don't need your help."

She just frowned and went to the bathroom. I immediately went to her purse and swiped a credit card out of her wallet.

* * *

Late September 1991
Back in the Counselor's Office

"So, what do you think the stealing was about?" the counselor asked.

"I was a compulsive thief for most of my teen years. One time when I shoplifted, I got caught. When my mother came to pick me up from juvenile hall, I felt like I had her complete attention for the first time. That was a new sensation. That stood out more to me than the fact that I had been picked up for shoplifting. I can count on one hand how many times my mother was really present for me, I mean completely in the moment with me."

"Go on," Kathryn encouraged. "It takes courage to talk about this. Don't stop."

"I think the reason I stole her credit card on this particular time when she came to see me in Baltimore, was that I didn't believe that she really wanted to help me," I explained. "I guess I was angry—very angry that now, after all these years, she was finally coming to get me. And even though she said she wanted to help me out, I felt it was really because *she* wanted help. Or maybe she just felt guilty because her friend's daughter had been murdered. It was like all of a sudden she woke up and she realized she had a daughter."

"Don't you think that if your mother could have done better, she would have done better? Or that perhaps she abandoned you because she had abandoned herself?"

I considered what Kathryn was saying, but the anger burned in my gut like acid, and I just couldn't feel any sympathy. "I've made excuses for her my entire life," I said. "The fact is, she looked the other way until it was convenient for her not to."

"I'm just trying to get you to look at your past in a new way."

I shrugged. "I guess that's your job."

"Well, I'm afraid our time is up," Kathryn said. "Will next week at the same time work for you?"

"I'm not sure. I mean, the wedding's pretty soon and I'm sure most of the major problems in our relationship have been resolved."

"So you are saying you won't be coming in anymore?"

"Maybe not."

"Whatever you think is best."

"Thanks for all your help, Kathryn."

"You're welcome. If you change your mind, I'm always here. You may sit here and rest as long as you like…I will be meeting my next client in the office adjacent to this one."

Adjacent, I thought. Why do shrinks talk like that? Still, I decided to take her up on the "resting as long as I like" thing. I filled my cup up with hot water from a hot and cold-water dispenser, and I put a tea bag in it. Chamomile. To calm my nerves.

All of a sudden, it started raining. I guess the combination of unexpected rain, and the appointment with the pre-marital counselor had me all choked up. Especially the stuff about my mother. How could she have not known what was happening to me? How could she have so artfully shut out the truth? Why did she allow me to wander the streets discovering the power of being a woman in all the wrong ways?

I tried a sip of the chamomile tea, hoping it would soothe me, but my nerves were shot and my emotions were raw and dangerously real.

Growing up, I viewed my mother as a passive, helpless victim, and I didn't want to be anything like her. She never seemed to be able to stand up to my stepfather, and because of this failure, her children became his private hostages. In rejecting my mother, I rejected the feminine.

Since my stepfather, who was a sex addict, appeared to have all the power, I equated sex with power. I would be a badgirl, since badgirls had all the power. *I created a superhuman femme fatale persona to protect me from feeling the pain of the hurt little girl within.*

The badgirl was nothing like Mom, who was powerless. The badgirl was all powerful, and very sexual. I believed that sex was my birthright. After all, young women in the fifties and sixties battled the puritanical myth that women were not supposed to enjoy sexual pleasure. And so, by being a sexually promiscuous woman, I was taking back what had been stolen from women like my mother.

I used sexuality over and over as a narcotic, and could not understand why I was filled with shame about my acting out. I wanted to be everyone's fantasy. I viewed myself with a double consciousness. I had this sense of always looking at my self through the eyes of men. I stood outside of myself watching. Split off from my real, authentic self, I could not feel the pain of my inner child.

While goodgirls were passive victims, badgirls enjoyed sex and were evil. I developed this persona to take control. Similarly, I used prostitution to take back control over my sexuality. I believed that the world of the sex industry offered the easy way out, a shortcut to power and control. *It was a shortcut that almost cost me my life.*

chapter twenty-two

Patrick and I drove down Market St. in downtown San Diego. Up ahead of us, some of San Diego's finest had pulled over a woman dressed in blue jeans and a ragged pink tee-shirt that said "Hollywood" in gold letters.

"Get her," shrieked Patrick.

His instant anger and hair-trigger reaction frightened me.

"Scum of the earth!"

"You don't even know that woman, Patrick," I said, feeling slightly nauseated.

"She's a god-damned hooker. What more do I need to know?"

I slid down into my seat. There was no way I could tell my soon to be husband about my past.

I don't know what's going on with Denise. Every time I talk to her, all she can focus on is going on the Phil Donahue show. And then she'll talk about setting up a threesome with some guy for five hundred bucks. If you ask me, it's all a big lie. Her life. Of course, she probably thinks the same thing about my life, and especially my upcoming marriage. Ever since I told her I couldn't invite her to the wedding, things just haven't been the same.

Patrick doesn't want me to hang around her anyway. He doesn't exactly understand my need to associate with ex-hookers. Only I'm not so sure she's really an ex-hooker. But he doesn't need to know that. If he found out that I was associating with a woman pretending to be an ex-hooker he would never let me into the doors of the Catholic Church. And he would certainly never allow me to pray, during the wedding ceremony, in front of a statue of the Virgin Mary, while a blonde, blue-eyed soloist performed angelic music. After all, I would then truly be damaged goods.

In the meantime, there was still hope. I could shape myself into the perfect bride. My sordid past would mean nothing juxtaposed with my perfected self. After all, my hair was dyed nearly platinum. I was now wearing a perfect set of acrylic nails. The area above my lip had been waxed, as well as my bikini line. Every part of me had been exfoliated, tweaked, plucked, and shaven to near perfection. Not a root, or a hair, or a nail bed exposed. The only problem was that this perfection was very short lived—about two days. Max.

The fleeting nature of my artificially constructed perfection was brought home to me when I had stopped off at a 7-11 convenience store on my way to the Sex Industry Survivor's meeting at the jail. In pursuit of a sugar high, I was standing in line to purchase candy bars and Twinkies. I knew I shouldn't be buying these items. There were only a few weeks remaining until my wedding and I still had more weight to lose if I wanted to fit into that size 7 dress. And then there it was. The cover of *Sports Illustrated* Swimsuit issue.

How could I ever measure up? At least I'd never stooped to getting fake breasts, I told myself. Then I drove off in my white 1988 Pontiac Firebird and I bit into a Twinkie which I hoped would quench my sense of nervousness and anxiety. I glanced down at my fire engine red nails. Damn if I hadn't broken a nail.

Once more, I wondered where Denise was. And I thought about Patrick calling that girl the scum of the earth. I felt frightened. I can't lie. All of a sudden I thought about what my mother said, about how I was "trying too hard to fit a round peg into a square hole." Maybe I wasn't marrying Patrick for the right reasons. Maybe, because of my past, I was jaded, and incapable of expressing real love.

I did know, as I finished off the second Twinkie, that I was really looking forward to my visit to the jail. When I went on the "inside," as they called it, something shifted in me. I felt like I was doing something good. I was showing them that they did have choices. This gave me a sense of peace that was new to me.

I pulled my Firebird into the jail parking lot. It felt strange to be there without Denise, or Joanne, the founder of Sex Industry Survivors Anonymous. I had never been to Los Colinas on my own. At least not as a panel leader. This time, I walked unescorted through the inside of the jail to reach the meeting place.

Although alone, I felt the presence of many unseen eyes upon me. Indeed, as I cut through the center of the jail compound, I noticed a camera attached to the top of a barbed wire fence. The jail authorities, as well as the women in the yard, were watching every move I made. I cut across what was supposed to be the jail lawn, a patchwork of green and mostly dull brown, and walked into the library/classroom where we were now holding the meeting.

I had already rehearsed what I was going to tell the inmates. I had myself pretty charged up by the time I entered the small classroom. The only problem was that it didn't look like many women were going to be showing up. Maybe there was a good Oprah episode on TV.

Finally, a female deputy poked her head into the room. "They'll be here in five minutes. One of them got rolled up."

"Rolled up?"

"Locked down," the deputy explained. "We put them in their cage and when they can behave we let them back out."

There was a glee in the deputy's eye that made me nervous. "Thanks," I said. "I'll just wait right here for them."

Finally, the group arrived, and I started into my pitch. "My name's Juliet, and I'm a sex industry survivor. I've got four years of clean time and I haven't turned a trick in ten years. It's the first transaction that sets up the addiction."

"What you mean, first transaction?"

"Hi—could you please tell me your name?" I asked.

"I'm Tia, addict, and let me tell you something—on a good night, I best be havin' a first transaction, or I'm fixin' to starve to death."

Undaunted, I continued to carry the message. "Yes, well, I want to explain that this is an addiction, a disease."

"I'm addicted to the drugs, all of us is, not the mens," Tia said. "They's just a means to an end."

I nodded in Tia's direction to let her know I understood where she was coming from. "I believe that it's an addiction to the sex industry," I explained. "And that if I get started with it, I can't stop. Is there anyone here who has had that experience?"

No one said a word.

"Is there *anyone* here who wants out of prostitution?" I ventured.

A diminutive blonde somewhere in her early twenties raised her hand. "I do."

"What's your name?" I immediately asked.

"Loretta…my name's Loretta and I've been into the life since I was fourteen. My mother got me into it. We were hitchhiking and this truck driver said he would give us a ride all the way to Tennessee. My mom told me what to do. She had to talk me through it. I've been in it so long I can't see another way. I think I had a run-in with that serial killer; the one who is killin' all the prostitutes. He tried to strangle me with a cord, but I got away. I tried to talk to the cops about it—do you think they cared? It didn't matter to them that I could've died."

"Do you think the cops are involved with the murders?" I inquired.

"I really couldn't say about all that, but I know one thing, the police sure look the other way when a hooker winds up in a dumpster." Loretta sighed. "I've dated cops."

I always thought that it was funny, or ironic anyway, that hookers called tricks their "dates."

"The ones in vice are the worst," Loretta complained. "They just want to get as much free sex as they can."

The women all nodded.

"I know what I'm going to talk about next is unfamiliar to you, but try and keep an open mind," I said, feeling apprehensive about what I was going to ask them to do. But I knew how helpful this type of work had been for me, and so I forged ahead. "At one time, all of us were little girls. We each still have a little girl in us. I know this will seem strange, but for a moment, close your eyes, and try to picture the little girl you once were."

Several women groaned. I knew this was a bit much for most of them. Two Hispanic girls stared at me, their expressions tough, defiant. Then I saw Fantasy, Tia and Loretta close their eyes, and so after about a minute went by, I began:

"Now, I want you to imagine that you are the mother of a little girl. Now, picture this little girl out on the streets," I instructed. "What would you do if you saw that she was taking off with a stranger in his car, and you had no idea where they were headed?" I studied the inmates and some shifted uncomfortably in their seats. Several of the women seemed to be having difficulty breathing. "Now, before you answer this, just sit, and think about what I've asked."

But then one of the inmates, who, up until this point had not said a word, spoke up. "I would chain my daughter to a bed before I would let her go out there," she passionately announced.

"What's your name?" I asked.

"I'm Sue. My mom found out I was out there and she was really hurt. But when I get out of here, I'm going to get back into it; I already have men putting money on my books."

When the men put money on their books then the girls can buy cigarettes, candy, etc. It also means they owe the men sex when they get out of jail.

"Can I ask you a question, Sue?" I politely requested. She nodded. "If it wouldn't be okay for your little girl to be involved in the sex industry, and if it hurt your mother so badly to know you were in, why is it okay for *you* to be out there?"

Sue shrugged. "It's not that simple to get out of it."

"I did it—I got out," I said resolutely, with my head held high. "And you can all do the same thing; all you need is a little faith, and a little willingness."

"Well, you went to college," Fantasy said. "You started out with more, but, for us, well, we can't just walk away. Sometimes if it's all you know it's better than nothing."

"I know what Fantasy means," Sue commiserated. "I've been in jails so many times already I've lost count. I want to change, I really do. I'm scared though; when I get out I'm going to this recovery home. I might be safe when I'm in there, but like she was saying, this is all I've ever known. Deep down, I hate men. Doing what I do makes me hate them even more. And so I have to make them pay."

"That's right," Tia nodded. "That's just the way it is. You can't change anything. I mean it's nice you come out here, takin' time from your busy day and all to see us. But most of us are only here because we'd rather do this than fold laundry, and we're hopin' it'll make us look better to the authorities."

I didn't say anything for a minute. And then, in a real loud voice, trying to talk above the constant chatter and jail talk—flinging my words out there, so that I can almost see them floating above their heads, I said, "There is this thing called grace—grace, meaning that we all get a second chance. We can start over."

The women are looking at me like I'm crazy. Two of them are whispering and laughing in the back of the room. Again, I felt like no one was really listening. My words were floating high above them, suspended in the jail atmosphere. "Sometimes I don't know if any of you are listening to me."

"Yes, we are," said Fantasy. "We're listening to you. We just aren't sure if you believe what you're saying."

That night, alone in the condo, feeling rather raw and emotional as I often did after one of the meetings in the jail, I got my journal out of its hiding place. I had been keeping a journal since I was about fourteen. My sister Marie got me into it. I grabbed my favorite pen and began to write.

The clock was ticking. In less than 30 days I would be walking down the aisle. I was getting scared. Soon there would be no exit—no more escape hatches, no more affairs, no more Sex Industry Survivors Anonymous or Sex and Love Addicts Anonymous meetings where I would swear: NEVER AGAIN! After all, as soon as I got married, I would be cured of my tendency towards duplicity. I would no longer crave my cake and the desire to eat it too.

One thing I know for sure—I have learned that part of my brain—that part where a conscience is stored, is not working correctly, or perhaps was not adequately developed during my childhood. I have an under-developed sense of right and wrong. It is difficult for me to feel guilt and shame about having affairs. I need to find out why, and get past this.

In pre-marital counseling, the therapist had this to say about my behavior. "You are still acting like a teenager, running away, not communicating, being evasive." She went on to tell me that if we had children, they would turn out to be flower children, or hippies.

How ironic that I spent my teen years, and almost every summer of my life in the Haight-Ashbury (hippie spawning ground) where I tried to get the attention and love of my hippie/convict father. Maybe that shrink was right, but she really pissed me off.

In order to grow, to become completely whole, I had to identify my personal myths. I had to keep looking into the eye of the storm called sexual addiction. I am a psychological detective, exploring the goodgirl/badgirl myth. And so I held up a magnifying glass to my last acting out episode. I wanted to examine what happened, and what preceded and followed the event.

It was the night that the cops discovered me with a young man in an alley. My behavior that night was dangerous, not to mention highly risky. After all, attempting to have sex in a public place is not legal. I was not in control of this behavior. This behavior could have gotten me arrested, not to mention jeopardize my health, and of course, my marriage.

I had met Man B at my usual nightclub, Kix. On this particular evening, I was feeling desperate. I was going to end my affair with Man A—this time I was serious. He had rejected me for the last time. When I got a hold of him, I would let him have it.

But I never did see Man A. Instead, I saw Man B, looking very good, I had to admit. We made joyful eye contact across the room and a decision was made. I would have sex, one last time. We parked in an alley behind a large grocery store. Moments later, flashing police lights interrupted what was about to take place.

That night, I went home and experienced gut-wrenching humiliation. My double life was unraveling. But my pain was brief and swift as my keen addict mind came to a brilliant conclusion. I decided that experimenting with bisexuality might be a solution to my out-of-control sex life. After all, men certainly had not been a solution.

And so I went to a lesbian bar where women playing at being men shot pool or grinded their hips together on the dance floor. I mustered up some courage and asked a greasy haired black girl to dance. She said no. My fragile ego had not anticipated this and so I headed for the door.

My *addiction wasn't working for me anymore,* I thought, as I put my journal back into its regular hiding spot. I knew, deep down, that whatever I was going through with Man A, or Man B, was just another example of a lifelong pattern. And attempting to switch sexual preferences wasn't the solution either. I used sex and romance to hideout from life.

During my first marriage, I had affairs because I didn't want to be married. When that marriage ultimately ended in divorce, I had multiple affairs so that I would not have to grieve. When I sobered up from alcohol and drugs, I was able to abstain for a while, but then the promiscuous behavior resurfaced.

chapter twenty-three

October 1991

I met Denise downtown at the YMCA. She had started another Sex Industry Survivors Anonymous meeting and wanted me to help her run it.

"Great location," I said. We were standing in the lobby. The receptionist peered at us, curious.

"Yeah, well this was the only place in San Diego that was willing to have a meeting like this. Most places hung up on me when I tried to explain it to them," Denise told me.

"I bet. The sex industry is our city's dirty little secret."

"How about the *world's* dirty little secret," Denise replied.

I nodded, following her down the hall. "I'm glad you could find a room for another meeting."

"It wasn't easy, but the good girlfriend pulled through, two snaps up," she said, flipping her curly blonde hair behind her. It was her trademark.

"So where were you?" I asked. "You missed the panel at the jail. I had to tell the girls at the jail that you weren't feeling well."

"What do you mean where was I—didn't you see it?" Denise said.

"See what?"

"I went on the Phil Donahue show!" Denise said.

"You did it, you went on the Phil Donahue show?" I cocked my head to one side. "But I thought you—"

"Say it," Denise said, her tone defiant. "You thought I relapsed. I already told you that I called an escort service two weeks before I went on the show."

"You went on National Television saying you weren't in the sex industry?"

"Yes. I said I'd been out of it for a year."

I shook my head, disgusted. "How could you do that?"

She placed her hands on her hips. "You're the one who can't stop having affairs."

"What does that have to do with going on TV and saying you're a reformed hooker when you aren't?"

"Depends on what you mean by reformed," Denise snapped back.

"What are you talking about?" I asked.

"All I need is the desire to leave the sex industry," Denise explained. "I have a desire—and so that means I'm reformed."

"But why would you purposefully misrepresent yourself?"

"Misrepresent. Isn't that some shit? Like you've never misrepresented yourself."

"Not on television."

"Like I said, all I need is a *desire* to get out. And I have that, I really do. But something just keeps pulling me back in."

A thin, dark-haired woman wearing a large Ankh symbol walked in just then. "Is this the Sex Industry Survivors Anonymous meeting?"

"It sure is," Denise and I said in unison.

After the woman joined us at the table, I began the meeting. "I'm Juliet, sex industry survivor."

"Hi, Juliet," Denise said.

"Welcome to the first official meeting at the downtown, San Diego YMCA," I said. "The purpose of this group is to help us heal from the sex industry. The sex industry can leave its mark in many different ways. Even though I've been out of it for a long time now, I still try to control and manipulate men sexually. I get off on the power."

I frowned. Rain began to tap against the only tiny window in the room. Denise and the woman wearing the ankh symbol peered at me, waiting for me to go on.

"I'm about to get married yet I can't stop having affairs," I continued. "I believe I'm locked into certain things because of my past. That's all I have for today. Thanks for letting me share."

"Thanks for sharing, Juliet. My name is Denise, and I'm a recovering prostitute."

"Hi Denise," I said.

"I guess I'll tell a little about myself," Denise said. "I almost relapsed—I tried to score some rock cocaine, but the dealer wasn't home, and when I left his house I couldn't find my car. I walked up and down the street, convinced it was stolen. I was just so obsessed with scoring that I had forgotten where I parked my car.

"Anyway, when I finally found it, I made a choice not to use, or turn a trick to get more rock. I don't want to die like the forty-five women that have been found murdered."

I lightly drummed my fingers on the table. I noticed how the top of the table was peeling. I wondered if she was going to tell the group how she had gone to work for an escort service two weeks before appearing on the Phil Donahue show.

Probably not. Just like I hadn't mentioned to the Catholic priest that I was having an affair with an Italian Portuguese stereo salesman even as I signed the papers swearing to eternal fidelity to my rageaddict recovering alcoholic fiancé.

How could either one of us admit to the truth—that our addiction to the sex industry had changed us into dishonest, self-willed people at odds with the world? We had become experts at manipulating the truth. So much so that we learned to believe our own lies. I tried to refocus my attention on what Denise was saying.

"The insanity of my latest experience has made me willing to make this program work. I'm just going to have to accept that I'm not going to make the same kind of cash I used to make from hooking it," Denise said. "Part of being in the life is the game of looking the best you possibly can out there. I always thought I had to have everything perfect. My underwear. My hair. And now I see that was all part of the game. Being that perfect woman. Everything so that I could be the perfect ho'. Now I'm willing to just be real."

Finally, it was the new woman's (the one wearing the Ankh symbol) turn to share. "Hi. My name is Chantelle, and I'm proud to say that I'm a recovering prostitute. I started into the life when I was married. We were living in Boston at the time. There was this man who wanted to go out with me. He offered me $300 to go to bed with him. I wound up leaving my husband because he was abusive—so $300 sounded like a lot to me. In the beginning, I was going with millionaires who owned yachts in the Boston Harbor. I was wearing mink stoles and eating in fancy restaurants."

Chantelle made eye contact with Denise and I, and then she continued. "It was 1975; I was 19. As time went on I was introduced to drugs. That's when my prostitution slid from being a call girl in elegant places to the massage parlors, and then to the street corner."

Denise and I smiled at her, attempting to reassure her and let her know she was not alone. We had seen our game change on us too. Buoyed up from the strength that comes from one addict talking to another, Chantelle continued to tell us about her descent from glitzy call girl to street ho'. "It happened quickly—say within a few months. Anybody that shoots drugs knows the story. I ended up on the streets, standing on the corner, turning tricks constantly; I mean I worked. I stayed there seven, eight days a week, 25 hours a day. My life became a living hell. I was gang raped and brutalized and held at knifepoint."

Even though Chantelle did look pretty torn up, I could see that she had once been a very beautiful woman. *So much for prostitution being a "victimless" crime,* I thought.

Chantelle sighed before she spoke again. "And then twenty years went by," she said wistfully. "One time I was with a trick—I was about 39—he was younger. When I wouldn't go to bed with him, he ripped my blouse off and threw me on the bed. He was a body builder so he was very strong. He held my arms down and pulverized my face, and beat me half to death. I went crazy—I went to grab a knife. There was no problem on my part; I would have killed him. You can believe that. And so I wound up in jail for attempted murder. Somehow, the charges were dropped. That's where I met you guys. The Sex Industry Survivor's meeting came into the jail. Denise and Joanne carried the message to me."

"That's right girl," Denise interjected.

"Now I'm dying—I have AIDS and Hepatitis C. I'm 46 years old and I'm dying." Chantelle slouched into the chair. For the first time I could see that her complexion was pale, too pale. "There are a lot of us that are dying. I have two friends with Hepatitis C, another with AIDS."

She managed a weak smile and I noticed she was missing quite a few of her teeth. To make a long story short, she wasn't in the best of shape. The sex industry was slowly killing Chantelle. The sex industry always kills, one way or another. *This sure ain't no*

"Pretty Woman," script, I thought.

When the meeting ended, Denise and I sat in the empty room.

"Listen," Denise said. "There's something else I need to tell you."

"Yeah," I said. "What is it?"

"I relapsed—not just with working," Denise admitted. "I did use. It was when I was looking for another hooker to go on the Phil Donahue show. I got triggered. I was on Market St. and I found a girl who said she would be on the show. But then she was about to use, and I used too."

"What did you use?"

"Crack cocaine."

"And then when did you do the show?"

"The next day," Denise replied candidly.

"Jesus," I said.

"Yeah, well, I'm clean now."

"How long," I started to ask, but changed my mind. Instead, I said, "I wish I could have gone on the show. I just didn't want to jeopardize my marriage."

"Hey, I didn't relapse because you couldn't be on the show," Denise reassured me.

"I know, but if I had gone on the show you wouldn't have been looking for that other girl," I said.

"I did what I did because I'm an addict," Denise said. "I'm not sure if I can change. I'm trying to, I really am…"

"I know Denise, I know."

In a rare display of emotions, Denise began to cry. Soft summer rain pelted against the windows and I put my arms around Denise.

My father called and told me he couldn't come to the wedding. Said he hasn't been out in the public, other than for court appearances, for many years. He claimed that even going to the store terrified him. "I do love you though," he said.

"Yes," I said. But I couldn't say anything more meaningful than that. I just felt a sense of emptiness. I guess I just hadn't forgiven him yet.

All my life I had been looking for a tangible sign that my father loved me. I considered attendance at my wedding to be symbolic of my father's love for me. One more time I felt an ache in my heart, and a raw gaping emptiness in my gut. My daddy hunger kicked in.

I believe most prostituted women have this daddy hunger. Some of them were raped by their daddies, abandoned by their daddies, ignored by their daddies, or ridiculed by their daddies. And so we have this daddy hunger.

When I was only nine months old, my father ran off with our sixteen-year-old babysitter and he never looked back. As a teen, I made several attempts at re-uniting with my father, but his wife did not want children around. And so he would drop me off at the homes of strangers, or at the Greyhound Bus Station in San Francisco.

If he had been paying closer attention to his underage daughter maybe, just maybe I wouldn't have made some of the choices I made. Of course, when you are locked up all the time like my father was, it's just about impossible to be a parent. Maybe one day I would forgive my father and it would probably happen the minute I chose to take complete responsibility for my past. But I wasn't there yet.

On my way home from the meeting, I drove through my old neighborhood. I was feeling sentimental, because I knew in a couple of months, right after the wedding, we would be moving to Ventura. I had grown to love San Diego, especially downtown San Diego, where I had lived for several years before I moved in with Patrick. I navigated the car down B Street, the part where the hills dip suddenly downward and you can see a panoramic view of the city for about one block and then it disappears.

Not to far from this neighborhood was where Denise had relapsed with that hooker who she had been trying to recruit for the Phil Donahue show. I thought of how she had cried at the end of our Sex Industry Survivor's meeting. It was one of about two times I had ever seen her cry.

A week later I was going over my wedding list. The phone rang. "Hello?"

"Juliet?"

"Yes, this is Juliet."

"It's Denise."

"Hey you. Glad you called. I was just sitting here trying to firm up wedding plans. I'm really sorry I couldn't invite you—you understand, Patrick just wouldn't like it."

"No, don't worry about it. I didn't call about that. I'm just having problems staying sober, in every area. You know what I mean?"

"I'm sorry. What can I do?"

"I need some money." She paused, and then continued her soliciting. "Not much, just enough to—"

"Just enough to buy more drugs?"

"I just have to get well, you understand."

"I can't, Denise," I said swiftly.

"I promise," she pleaded, her voice becoming more desperate. "I'll get it back to you next week."

"No—I can't."

"You've got to help me. Just this one time."

"No really, I can't. And I really don't even think you should call me anymore. I don't think we're going down the same path anymore."

"I thought you were my friend—how could you do this to me," Denise whined.

"This is ridiculous."

"You just want to make sure I don't show up at your wedding. That's what all this is about."

"This has nothing to do with my wedding."

"This has everything to do with your wedding, girlfriend. Your fancy Catholic all dressed in white wedding. And you know something, it's the biggest lie you've ever told."

"You could be right Denise, you really could be."

"If I'm so right than why don't you want me to call you anymore?"

"I can't hang out with you when you're using. You've got to understand that."

"It's like that, is it?"

"Please don't call me anymore."

"Look, can't you just give me ten bucks, that's it, that's all I need," she begged.

"No, Denise, I'm sorry, I can't."

On the other end of the line, I heard the sound of her slamming the phone down, and I just sat there, and a deep sadness flooded over me. I had wanted to be her friend, but that was impossible now. And yet, she had changed my life. If I had never met Denise, I would have locked my secret deep, deep inside of me for an entire lifetime.

chapter twenty-four

Mid October 1991
Santee, California
Los Colinas Women's Jail

Female inmates from Los Colinas waved themselves with makeshift paper fans. Sweat rolled down red, swollen faces. It was one of the hottest Indian summers San Diego had experienced in decades. It was bad enough to be incarcerated, but in this heat it must surely be hell. A few of them frowned at me as I walked, dressed in my cool professional attire, through the center of the jail compound. I can see why they resented me. After all, I was free to walk in, and then free to walk out. Taking complete advantage of this freedom, I eavesdropped.

Inmates clustered around picnic tables told each other stories. Their stories made them forget all the close calls and near brushes with death. Their stories took them way beyond this place, above the barb-wired fences, and into a fantasy world. When they got out this time, they assured one another, they would make their hustle work.

When I walked into the library, Darlene, the counselor, looked surprised to see me. I noticed she had started to set the room up for the meeting. "Hi Juliet; I wasn't sure if you were going to be here or not today."

"Hi Darlene. I like to keep my commitments," I said, and began to shape the plastic chairs into a circle.

"I'm glad," Darlene said. "The women look forward to this meeting."

I put the last chair in place and looked up. "I also came to say goodbye."

"Goodbye—really, why?" Darlene said.

"I'm getting married in thirty days, and we're moving to Ventura."

"Congratulations, Juliet, that's wonderful. And thank you so much for doing all this. You've set a great example for the women."

"You don't have to thank me. Coming out here has been an incredible gift. I should thank you, and the women here."

She smiled, and in a more serious tone, said, "I heard you and Denise had a falling out."

"I guess you could call it that," I responded softly, as I watched a male deputy escorting six women into the library. They all smiled and waved at me. This warmed my heart instantly.

"So," Darlene whispered, "what really happened between you two?"

I watched the women fill into the circle. I really didn't want to answer the question. I felt responsible for the demise of my friendship with Denise. And if it had not been for Denise and Joanne, there never would have been a meeting here at all. What other hookers had bothered to start a support group in jail? Who was I to judge her? I just couldn't be friends with her right now. It was too confusing.

"She relapsed," I said, feeling as if I were betraying her even as the words were coming out of my mouth.

"She relapsed?

I nodded.

"If what you are saying is true she won't be able to come back to this meeting until she has at least six months clean time," Darlene said.

"It's true, that's why she isn't here."

"I see."

"Well, I better get the meeting started."

And so I began to tell them my story. How I had an addiction to the life, to controlling men, to using my sexuality to gain power over men. "For me, it was progressive. In the end, I wanted five sugar daddies instead of one. One wasn't enough, just like with the drinking—one drink wasn't enough. I was powerless. And if I hadn't gotten sober from drugs and alcohol, I never would have been able to talk about my former life as a prostitute."

All of the inmates actually seemed to be listening to me. It wasn't often that I felt I had their undivided attention. But then the pain started up, just like it always did. *Damn. Why did it always have to hurt so much?* I fought to keep the tears from coming. But my emotions were just too strong.

"You go girl," said a large black girl. "Don't even bother holding it back."

"I'm sorry," I said, attempting to wipe my tears away.

"Don't say you sorry," said the same black girl.

Fantasy, the nineteen year old who now appeared to be *very* pregnant, got up from the circle and went to get me a Kleenex. I accepted it and after dabbing my makeup smeared eyes, went on. "I guess the reason it hurts so much to talk about it is that I kept it all a secret for so long. The first time I started talking about it was when I came to see you guys. But they say the truth shall set you free, and I know it has worked that way for me. Each time I talk about my past, it's easier, less painful the next time. And I'm actually starting to like myself, especially when I look at how far I've come. I've been out of the industry for ten years. I have a job as a technical writer in the computer industry.

"Because of my sobriety in all areas, including drugs, alcohol, and the sex industry, I am free to pursue my goals and dreams. I have choices…options. And most important of all—I have a connection with God today. I want you all to find what I have found. So, what about you guys. Any of you want to talk today?"

"My name's Renee. I don't know if I want to quit. I'm not sure I see anything wrong with it. But when I'm on the curb, I never stand; I always walk, because I feel ashamed." She looked around at the other women and then quickly added, "But I like the money…the freedom."

"Thanks for sharing, Renee," I said.

"My name's Tasia. And I'm not sayin' whether I'm a sex survivor, or whatever you call it, or not. N' fact, I was just outside talkin' to my home girls. Man they kin' take this heat. Anyway, I was tellin' my home girls that I like the streets cuz I can turn a trick and then kick back and hit the pipe or whatever. What happened with me is I started workin' the curb—you know—then I got into jackin' the tricks. You know; it was like, excitin'…I liked it."

"Explain 'jack' again," I said, and the women cracked up.

"Oh you know, that's when you steal from the tricks," Tasia quickly explained. "You jack em up. Believe me, it has it's ups and downs, you know."

"What are the downs?" I asked.

"I guess when the other ho's be lookin' down on you. Like there was this neighborhood girl who gives head to get crack, but then she be like, lookin' down at me and calling me a slut. She a slut, too."

I paused for a moment and then said, "That's just her denial. Does anyone else want to share?"

"My name is Sarah."

"Hi Sarah," I said.

"I've been doing this for fifteen years," Sarah continued. "I don't mind it. But see, the thing I like is freedom. I don't know what else I would do. I mean you have a skill, you work with computers—but this is all I'm good at."

"You could go to school, Sarah," I said, trying to encourage her. "You could even request job training while you're in here."

"Job training?" Sarah said doubtfully.

"Yes, learn some new skills," I persisted. "Even though I work full-time, I'm taking writing classes at night so I can get this certificate. There are all kinds of ways to get more education."

"I doubt my pimp would appreciate my trying to get an education," Sarah said, declining my suggestion outright. "Besides, I like what I do. What I don't understand is how the johns can hate me so much for being a hooker."

Sarah crossed her arms tight and bent her head. "I had one guy rape me anally for six hours," she said in a soft whisper. "He was arrested for raping all these other women. When he was doing it he kept telling me that I was just another whore and I deserved it. But what else can I do? Like I said, I don't have any other skills. At least when I'm a hooker I can work whenever I want to. I can check into whatever hotel I want, order room service, and get away from people," Sarah looked up, uncrossed her arms, and sat up straight. "When I'm in my hotel room, I'm calling the shots and I'm free."

Sarah paused. She looked through the only window in the room; two tiny squares at the top of the door. "The only problem is, lately, every time I turn a trick I get ripped off by some gang member. So I just got a pimp and he helps make sure I eat and sleep. I bought him a car and clothes and he's only put twenty dollars on my books." She shrugged. "I guess every job has its drawbacks. Besides, I can't do some nine to five deal. I need my freedom."

I just smiled and waited for the next woman to share. It was sad the way women in the sex industry always wanted to talk about how they were so free. They needed to believe in their own freedom desperately, otherwise they would not be able to continue in the life. They were, in fact, not free. They were slaves to their own limited beliefs, such as the idea that being a whore was all they were worth. Slaves to their addictions. *Slaves to the cyclic world of the sex industry. Do drugs to be able to do the work. Do the work to do the drugs. Then do the time.*

The next woman who shared was pretty torn up.

"I'm not a prostitute," she insisted, "I'm an addict. Oh, I know I might have slept with men to get drugs, but that's because I always had drug dealer boyfriends. But I ain't no ho."

"What are you in here for?" I asked, even though we weren't supposed to.

"Solicitation. But it was a set up," she insisted.

"I believe you," I said. "Look, it's possible to get out of all this. You just have to want it. You have to want it more than you want anything else. You have to be willing to change everything. I did it, and so can you."

A Hispanic woman in her forties scowled, her tattooed arms crossed across her chest. "Maybe for you, being white and all. You might have a chance. But in the hood' all there is for us is the curb, or joining a gang. Because of the gangs, you know, like the Bloods, or the Crips, today, it's all about the crack cocaine. And sister, that stuff has created a world of monsters. Homeboys will snuff you out or jack you up so quick and then laugh about it. The worse they treat the women the more macho they think they are. I want to get out of all of it but it isn't that easy. You get branded."

"What did you say your name is?"

"I didn't. You might as well just call me by booking number since I've been in and out of here so many times."

The women in the circle laughed. I didn't laugh, however. I thought her comment was sad, and so true for most of them. Many of the inmates were just about "institutionalized," or so used to being in the system that it really wasn't any big deal one way or the other.

"I don't want to call you by your booking number," I said. "And I don't want you to call yourself by that either. None of you have to come back here. Don't you think it's really about choices? You can make some new choices, and then maybe, just maybe, you'll have different outcomes."

The Hispanic woman crossed her arms even tighter so that one of her tattoos almost looked like a swastika. "You don't really get it, do you? Once you get branded, you can't just walk away. It ain't that simple, and for some of us, it's safer in here." She straightened her arm for my examination. "These are my gang tattoos. They mean I've been jumped into my gang. When I get out of here, I belong to them. They share me. Then I go out and make money for them, and that's the way it is."

"What would happen if you tried to leave the gang?" I asked.

"I'm dead," she said. "Just like that, and after the homeboy pulled the trigger, his dogs would laugh and call him a man."

I believed her. My chest felt tight and the library suddenly seemed really warm. It was getting to be that time. I had to tell them that I wouldn't be coming back. I cleared my throat and said, "As most of you women know, I'm about to be married."

"You go girl," one woman said. "Congratulations."

"I guess that's the good news. The bad news is that I won't be coming back here, so, unfortunately, this group won't be meeting anymore."

"You aren't coming back?" Fantasy asked.

I shook my head. "I wanted to tell you women how much you've meant to me."

"You too, Juliet," Tasia said. "But maybe one day we'll see you in here."

"No, I don't think so. I haven't seen this place since the early eighties when I was arrested for drinking and driving—and that's a direct result of my sobriety. But I'd really like to see some of you at meetings when you get out."

We all said the Lord's Prayer. A couple of the women gave me a hug, even though it was against the rules. I said my final goodbyes to all of them, and walked out of the library. I didn't look behind me because I cared about these women and I knew that the odds were pretty high that I might not see any of them ever again.

I moved quickly through the courtyard and strode into Darlene's office. She thanked me again and told me I would need to turn in my badge at the front reception area. As I walked through the courtyard towards the reception area, Fantasy, one of the few inmates who had attended the meetings regularly, waved at me. I smiled and waved back. The sun lowered over the courtyard, and the stories continued. Three Latino women had found the only patch of shade at the side of one of the housing units. Despite the unrelenting heat, they appeared so carefree, so nonchalant, as they chomped on the chocolate cookies and Doritos they just bought from their jail commissary.

What difference had my visits made here? Maybe not all that much, to them anyway, but to me, the visits to Los Colinas Women's jail had changed my life. Listening to their grim, violent stories had made me eternally grateful that I was no longer involved in the sex industry.

If I spoke with the women from Los Colinas ten years from now, I wondered how many of them would be able to say the same thing. Since there is a high mortality rate for those who are sex workers as well as drug addicts, the reality is that I might be the only survivor. But until then, at least they had the illusion of freedom and control over the men who purchased them.

One thing that intrigued me about working with the prostitutes in the women's jail is how skillful they had become at shutting out reality. For example, they said that walking down the boulevard, or the track, made them feel important. They had the feeling of being a star in their own movie. They felt like they were "it," in control and super powerful.

Even when their fantasy world was shattered by rape, murder and the countless other assaults made on sex workers every day in every city, these incarcerated women still wanted to cling to the romantic perception that out there on the streets they were a star. And yet the ever-increasing violence against women is far from glamorous. In one meeting I heard one woman talking about hookers being buried alive with rocks stuffed in their mouths. Then in the next breath, the same person would proclaim, "at least sex workers had their freedom."

Our denial made us believe we were "somebody" as we walked the boulevard. And it is our denial that makes us believe that we are special to tricks, pimps, or anyone else associated with the sex industry. But I had seen the truth, the low-down dirty truth about where the addiction takes prostituted women. And I knew that I had been given a precious gift. The gift of sobriety. The gift of healing. The gift of life. I was beginning to be healed. Not cured but healed. I was healing because I was telling the truth about my past. I was integrating my shadow. I was revealing parts of myself that I had fought to submerge. I was working at becoming whole.

I stood outside of the door that connected the inside of the jail with the outside. I looked up into a closed-circuit camera aimed right at me. I smiled, waved, and pressed the buzzer. But before I left Los Colinas, I got one last whiff of that awful jail smell: a combination of Lysol and the unmistakable aroma of human desperation. I found myself holding my breath.

I walked by three inmates. Each of them stopped walking, bowed their head, and looked down to the ground. This was a jail rule; it was easier to control the inmates that way. I passed three women in the holding tank who were waiting to be booked in. Then I waited outside of a small room where I pressed yet another buzzer. The guard on the other side nodded, and the door before me slid slowly open. I walked through the gray metal room into the reception area. I signed a sheet and returned my visitor's badge.

"See you next time," she said.

I just smiled, and walked out of the institution. *My name is Juliet, and I am a sex industry survivor,* I thought, as I heard the jail door lock behind me. And maybe I didn't always love my "day job" as a technical writer, but at least I was a professional, and I was, for a woman, well paid for my abilities. I had come a long way. Hell, in my own way maybe I could even dare call myself a success. For years I had waited for my mother and father to acknowledge how far I had come. Perhaps it was more important that *I knew* how far I had come.

As I walked away from the jail and towards my car, I felt a mixture of emotions ranging from bittersweet sadness, pride, and another state of mind quite unfamiliar to me. I felt triumphant. I was one of the lucky ones. *I had made it out of the sex industry alive, and now I had a chance to help others get out.* Maybe there really was hope for me, and hope for other survivors. All I had to do was be willing to help another survivor, and who knows what kind of miracles might take place. I was beginning to know what it felt like to make a difference in other women's lives, and I liked it.

chapter twenty-five

The wedding was planned for the beginning of December. Since it was now the end of October, I was running out of time. I simply had to get all the wedding details in place. One morning, my mother called. I thought she would ask about the wedding, but she seemed to just want to find out gossip about my sister.

"No," I said. "I haven't heard anything about Marie. But my wedding plans are coming along great. The colors are going to be beautiful. I'm going with blues and—"

"Well I think she's drinking again," my mother interrupted, obviously oblivious to what I had just said.

"Mom—the colors—I said the colors are going to be beautiful."

"Yes, I heard you. It's been almost a week since I've heard from her. Has she called you?"

"No, Mom, I haven't heard from her. Did I tell you about our wedding vows? They are going to be beautiful. I wrote them myself, and—"

"I told her she should get a job."

"Oh mother, why? She's a mom; that's her job. Why can't you just accept her the way she is?"

"I raised four kids and managed to work full time."

"Yeah," I said. *And you looked the other way while your husband sexually abused your two daughters. You drank and took those damned pills and looked the other way. Then your daughters became your slaves, desperate to keep you from committing suicide.*

"I just don't know why she can't manage to get herself together."

"She's an alcoholic, Mom."

"You are too, and you've done just fine."

I worked as a hooker to pay my way through college, but other than that, I did great. "It's been harder for her; after all—she got most of it."

"Most of what?" my mother said.

I paused. "Most of the sexual abuse."

"Oh, for God's sakes, not that again. Why can't you just forget about all that?"

"Forget about it…why can't I forget about it? Mom, that kind of thing stays with you for a lifetime."

"I would think you would have other things on your mind. Like your wedding plans."

"But I *have* been trying to talk to you about wedding plans and you aren't hearing a word I'm saying," I shot back at her. "All you can talk about is Marie."

"Well, I just had surgery and she didn't even think to call."

"I'll call her for you mom, is that what you want to hear?"

"Yes, and then call me right away, would you?"

"Yes, Mother," I said, and then I hung up the phone.

Fires had blazed all through South Central Los Angeles. The city had become a war zone. If only this were a horror movie, I thought. But it wasn't. This was real—the end result of riots sparked off when four police officers were acquitted of a certain crime. The cops had brutally beaten a suspect and the whole thing had been videotaped.

I turned off the television, but I could not stop thinking about the brutal images I had just witnessed. I had seen the very same kind of rage and bigotry when my fiancé would exhibit what can only be described as blind rage. Perhaps marrying a rageaholic/recovering/alcoholic/ex-smoker with a possible heart condition was my own form of self-inflicted punishment for my crimes of the past.

I wondered if the riots were an omen that I really wasn't supposed to be getting married. Patrick and probably the rest of the members of the Christian right-wing thought the riots, fires and other natural disasters that had been taking place across our nation were signs that the end times were coming. It all had something to do with one of the books in the Bible, the "Book of Revelations," and the fact that the new millennium was just around the corner.

Not wanting to think so apocalyptically, I tried to reassure myself. *Everything will be okay,* I told myself. *It will be a big beautiful wedding and I will be a classic bride, and we will ride off into the sunset.* And perhaps the timing of the riots really wasn't such a bad thing, after all. People might not want to travel during the riots, and that might not be such a bad thing, since the guest list was getting a little too top heavy. Since, as usual, my father wasn't contributing anything financially for the wedding, and each dinner plate was now up to $20.95, the mounting costs were definitely a concern.

I tried to ignore the nagging sensation of truth residing in the back of my mind that kept telling me that the cost of the wedding plate really wasn't what I ought to be looking at. After all, the vast cultural, religious, and political differences between my future groom and I would be the far more serious issues facing me after we made our triumphant march down the aisle. But I was going through with this. Come hell or high water—or riots in LA—I was going through with this.

Last Week of October 1991
San Diego

I went downtown to the Sex Industry Survivors Anonymous meeting being held at the YMCA. Right away, Joanne, the founder, showed up.

"I heard you and Denise aren't speaking," she said to me. "She told me she wouldn't be here until you two can patch things up."

"That might be a while then," I admitted. "Did you know she isn't allowed to go back to the jail until she has six months clean again?"

"Did you tell people at Los Colinas that she wasn't clean?" Joanne asked.

I just looked at her. Was I supposed to have lied for her? *Apparently so,* I thought, as I followed Joanne into the small room. The big industrial size clock on the wall read 7:30. The meeting started at 8:00 p.m.

"You don't understand this deal do you?" Joanne said.

"I don't follow you," I commented, genuinely curious.

"It's about desire," she explained, folding her pudgy arms across her chest.

I sat down across from her at the table. "What's about desire?"

"All we need—all Denise needs—is a *desire* to quit the sex industry," Joanne said. "Just like in Alcoholics Anonymous; all that's required is a desire to quit drinking."

"I realize that," I said.

"Oh do you? Well then why'd you squeal on her?"

"I didn't squeal on her! I just told Darlene, the jail counselor, what *happened*. I told her that Denise had relapsed. I thought Denise's relapse would be too confusing for the women."

"You were the only one who was confused," Joanne said. "I guess you believe that *you've* never relapsed, is that it? Can you look me right in the eye and tell me you've never done anything that couldn't be considered a transaction?"

"A transaction?"

"That's right. A transaction. A trade. Sex for money. Or sex for something you need, like your rent paid."

I felt my face turning red. Several examples came quickly to mind. In each case, I had maneuvered, conned, and negotiated to get something that had benefited me materially.

"I thought so," she replied.

"But I didn't even say anything."

"You didn't have to," Joanne said. "Until you can get real with yourself, Juliet, there's something you need to know. You aren't any better than Denise, and I don't care if you were an exclusive call girl or a filthy crack ho'."

"I never said I was better than anyone."

"Your actions show that you do." Joanne leaned towards me, her facial expression intense. "Look, sometimes there's a gap between the desire to quit, and actually being able to quit. But that doesn't mean you shut that person out. Denise has come a long way you know. She brought that meeting to the jail."

I nodded. "I know that."

"The last time she was arrested, she weighed about ninety pounds," Joanne said. "She was practically dead. She was working the streets daily and acting in hardcore porn. I think she appeared in about 400 of them."

"Yeah," I acknowledged. "She told me about that."

"So the point is, Denise may have slipped but she didn't go down nearly as far as she used to."

"You're right," I said reluctantly. "I guess I hadn't thought about it like that."

"If Denise is out there, it's because her *addiction* has her," Joanne firmly stated. "She can't choose right now—she's lost the power of choice. Once you take that first transaction the addiction gets triggered."

I thought for a moment about how hard it had been for me, in my first few months of sobriety, to admit that I was an alcoholic. I guess they call it denial. And now, the same part of me was *still* fighting against the disease concept as applied to my addiction to the sex industry. I was judging Denise as somehow morally less superior to me because she kept relapsing. Instead of judging my friend, I needed to pray for her, and to also remember that AA slogan: "But for the Grace of God go I."

"Maybe I was being a little judgmental," I was forced to admit. "So, what happened for you? How did *you* finally get out of it?"

"I guess I finally reached a point where I came to the realization that there were some things money couldn't buy," Joanne said. "I figured out that what I was really trying to find in money was protection. But no matter how much money I got from working in the sex industry, I still never felt safe, just like I never felt safe in my childhood."

"I think I used money for the same thing," I said. "I believed If I could just get enough money, If I looked good on the outside, then no one would ever know how terrified I felt inside."

She paused for a moment before she spoke again, her voice wistful as she recalled early memories. "I remember there was one night I spent watching my father force my mother to wax the kitchen floor until like two in the morning. Then he made her *strip* the wax, and then *re-*do it, again and again until he decided it was clean enough. I don't think it could ever be clean enough for him. After all, according to him, she couldn't do anything right. She couldn't even talk on the phone without him criticizing every word she said."

Joanne grimaced, remembering. "Everything changed one Christmas. My father bought me a baby doll nightgown and he insisted that I model it for him. I'll never forget that time because it was the first time he came after *me* instead of my mother, and I knew she wouldn't be able to do a thing about it."

"My stepfather bought a nightgown like that for my sister," I said.

"You're damn lucky he didn't get *you* one," Joanne sputtered angrily. "One night my father came into my room, telling me that he was gonna tuck me in, but instead of tucking me in he grabbed my breasts. Then he told me that next time I better have on the baby doll nightgown. When I told him to leave he said that he was just trying to be a nice daddy."

I felt sick as I listened to her story. It sounded all too familiar.

"My father never would allow me to wear any jewelry, makeup, or sexy clothes to school. So after awhile, I wore one set of clothes to school, and then, once I got to school, I would change into a second set of clothes I kept in my locker. I was already learning to turn into someone else. But even though I dressed like the other girls, I still didn't feel like I fit in.

"I started developing before other girls, and I was smarter than most kids. So I felt different. Plus I started being able to predict things. That really used to freak my father out. Eventually, he moved out, and he stole everything we owned. But I was so glad he was gone I didn't care if we did have to eat rice and beans for dinner every night."

"What happened then?" I asked.

"A few months later a neighbor boy raped me," Joanne said somberly. "He told me that it was his job to bust all virgins so that the other men wouldn't have to bother. Between the rape and my father molesting me I started hating sex, I mean really *hating* it. It used to make me sick, like I'd get migraines or I'd feel like I was going to throw up. So what I did was I learned how to hypnotize myself during sex. I would just split off from myself, go into this other world, do you know what I mean?"

"Yeah, I do know," I said sincerely. "I call it the split, or my glass cage."

"I've heard you call it that," Joanne said. "Anyway, I learned how to abuse my body—which is what I believe prostitution is. At the age of fifteen, I started having sex with at least four to five guys a night. I never enjoyed it, but it made me feel like I could conquer what I thought of as my own sexual dysfunction. Becoming a whore was all about taking back control."

"Maybe that's why I did it too," I said, shaking my head. "I just never thought of it that way. I felt I had to be sexual even though I really didn't want to be. By the time I was sixteen I was completely out of control. I had no boundaries. No self-respect. So when I started charging for sex, I felt like at least I was calling the shots."

Joanne nodded, and gave me a look that told me she knew exactly what I meant. So much of what Joanne told me matched my own experience. Like Joanne, I had been sexually and emotionally abused by my male caretaker. Although bright and gifted in school, I, just like Joanne, learned early on that it was my appearance, not my intelligence that would be rewarded.

Another thing that I have noticed in talking with sexually addicted women, or those who have been in the sex industry, is that they often identify with the sexually addicted father, and reject the vulnerable, powerless mother. This is what I did, and I believe this is what Joanne did. We made a decision early on that our mothers had no power and that we did not want to be anything like them.

Our sexually addicted male caretakers had all say, all power, all control, and so of course they became our role models. Because we associated sex with power, we unconsciously emulated the very ones who had perpetrated against us. Thus the cycle that started with incest, led into sexual addiction, and ultimately led us into the sex industry was initiated.

"Is this the meetin' for hookers who don't wanna be hookers no more?"

"It sure is," Joanne and I chimed in unison.

"Well, my name is Mercy," she said, taking a seat. "And this is Linda," she said, pointing to the woman who had walked in with her.

"Hey," Linda said.

"I was going to turn a trick, but I came here instead. I heard you guys, that is, well you," Mercy said, pointing to me. "I heard you speak at Los Colinas women's jail. Some of the things you said kept floatin' back to me. Sometimes I have to look at my motives. Do I hang out with someone because I know he has money, or do I come here?"

"How long have you been in the sex industry?" I asked.

"Oh no," Mercy said, "It's not like that. I never was a hooker, it's her—my alter."

Joanne and I exchanged glances. "Your who?" Joanne asked.

"My other personality, Lynette," Mercy said. "She's the one who turns the tricks. I have two or three of these alters. I have multiple personality disorder."

Joanne nodded with authority. "It's very common in our line of work."

"Lynette told me that my parents were part of a satanic cult. She told me that there had been abuse—severe, constant, ritualistic sexual abuse, maybe even child pornography. She told me such horrible things," Mercy said, slouching in her chair. "They sacrificed animals, there was blood everywhere, blood and little children."

Then Mercy stopped talking. She straightened in her seat and folded her hands neatly, resting them on the tabletop. "Just ignore Mercy. She's a bad girl. I'm the good one of the bunch...I'm Tammy Lee."

"Hi, Tammy Lee," Joanne and I said, looking at each other, astonished.

"I'm not a prostitute. That's the other alter, Mercy. Our father used to sexually molest her, and then the next day he would act like nothing had happened. There was something wrong with her to make him want to do that. She was evil and bad. When I, that is, when she, turns tricks, it was just like when our father used to touch us down there."

"Do you feel like you split off from yourself when you, or when your alters turn the tricks?" Joanne asked.

"I just tune out," Mercy/Lynette/Tammie Lee said. "I remember once opening the door to this leased trick apartment and there was this 300-pound man. In he came with his amyl nitrate, asking me if I brought the pink garter belts he had specially requested at the agency."

She sighed deeply before she continued. "I had to pray in order to get through it. All I kept telling myself was that I was making money. The only problem is that I didn't want to live any more. I was thinking about suicide. When I got busted it was down on the stroll, on 52nd and El Cajon. This really mean cop made me have sex with him. Then he turned around and arrested me."

"It's getting worse and worse out there," Joanne said.

"It's like they hate us," Mercy said. "That's why I haven't been out there since I got out of jail this time. But Lynette keeps wantin' to pull me into it again."

"Our disease tells us that we should keep doing what we're doing, even though it's like putting a gun to your own head," Joanne said.

The downtown San Diego Sex Industry Survivor's meeting had a pretty good turnout. Present were Joanne, myself of course, then there was Mercy, who only counted as one even though she had multiple personalities, her friend Linda, and a young black girl.

"Would you like to share next?" I asked the woman who had come in with Mercy.

"I guess so, but I'm only here to keep my friend Mercy company. My name is Linda and I like what I do. I'm 33 and I've been a prostitute since I was seventeen. But I'm not on the streets anymore. I've got regulars, you know, sugar daddies."

A young black woman, no more than eighteen, said, "Oh, come on. Even if it's a sugar daddy, it's *still* the same thing. You gotta be what *he* want you to be and you aren't even your own self. I'm sick of it. I want to get out. But no one cares. Once I stood, in the rain, at a payphone, on hold with a runaway hotline I'd called two hours earlier. I didn't want to run away, but my mother was a heroin addict and one night she just threw me out. I was fifteen years old with a little plastic bag of clothes, walking down the boulevard all alone. I didn't know *nothin.'* A man drove by and told me he would help me. That's how I got started."

She lifted up her shirt and showed us a scar that covered her stomach. "A trick did this. I wish there was something else I could do."

"You just need to be street smart," Linda interjected. "You need to know what's up. I can tell whether or not a trick is a psychopath in an instant. Besides, like I said, I don't even need to work the streets. I can always get myself set up in a nice hotel room for at least a week.

"There was this one time though..." All of a sudden, Linda's demeanor became a little less aggressive, less boisterous. Even her tone of voice seemed softer. "Well, what happened is this crazy trick told me he was going to bury me alive. He took me to this lover's lane at 3 a.m. The only thing that saved me was that luckily, some couple drove up to make out. He had the shovel ready and everything. I guess that was his thing—burying women alive. But you know, that was just a one-time thing. Usually I can spot the weirdos right away."

My name is Juliet. I am a sex industry survivor. Is it possible for me to recover from the sex industry? I think it is. I'm finding that although it's quite painful, it's also courageous for me to totally admit to, and then to finally let go of, my dark ugly past. The more I keep talking about it, the less painful it is. And although I doubt whether or not I'll ever be able to forget what happened to me, I realize that at least I no longer need to be ashamed of it.

I mean it's not as if one day you wake up and say to yourself, "Oh, I'm going to be a whore." No. It's not like that at all. More likely, perhaps, a friend might one day casually mention a way to make money in such a way that it doesn't sound too bad. After all, there you are, angry, hurt, hungry, and desperate. Her offer sounds good at the time—an easy, quick solution.

But then the solution, over a period of time, winds up becoming your life. And then the life winds up taking over. First you'll become addicted to the fast, constant, easy money, then to the men, and ultimately you're addicted to the illusion of control. What at first sounds like a glamorous night out on the town, will, eventually, prove to be soul-destroying, self-destructive and for far too many, lethal.

For countless men and women who wind up trapped in the sex industry, prostitution becomes a way in which the sex worker re-enacts the incestuous experiences they experienced in childhood. Once a person becomes a victim of sexual abuse, he or she will often split off, or disassociate from their authentic, core self and inner being. I call this "The Split."

When the victim has reached this stage, something internal has shattered. Unless a survivor manages to become aware of just how deeply her consciousness has become thoroughly fragmented, only then can she have much hope for healing. Until then, she stands outside of herself, in limbo, watching her own life as if watching a movie. She will feel as though she's become homeless in her own body.

I had to admit I had an addiction to the sex industry. I had to take the first step and admit I was powerless. Once I take that first transaction, I become powerless over my addiction. If I continue to be a whore "spiritually," I will initiate a cycle of relapse, which will surely get progressively worse. In order for me to heal from the sex industry, I'm required to abstain from *any* sex related earnings or exchange.

The bottom line is that if I choose to remain a whore spiritually, I will return to the sex industry, sooner or later, in one fashion or another.

chapter twenty-six

December 1991
Mission Valley (Condo Land) a Neighborhood of San Diego

I sat on my living room couch. I was doing a crewel embroidery project, which pictured a bouquet of flowers. I was pretty sure that the whole thing would take at least another year. Presently, I considered embroidery a therapeutic pastime. With the wedding less than ten days away, I needed all the stress-relieving activities I could fine.

My grandmother had taught me to embroider when I was a teenager. My first big embroidery project was really quite ambitious—it was an entire tapestry complete with a built-in political statement. Across the bottom of that tapestry I had diligently stitched: EQUAL RIGHTS AMENDMENT, 1982. And then, on another edge, "THE RIGHT TO BE." In the middle of this tapestry I had stitched a large, multicolored kite. In an attempt at patriotism, I added red, white and blue stars and stripes on the top half of the kite.

I put the tapestry I was now working on (the one with the timid flowers) and remembered that time. Remembered my feminism. Remembered how strong my beliefs in feminism were back then. During the 70s, while still in my teens, I had been exposed to what was referred to as the second wave of the women's movement. I remembered how I even marched in a consciousness-raising group that was protesting violence against women.

The colors in my "EQUAL RIGHTS AMENDMENT, 1982" tapestry had been as passionate and alive as my anger. Anger that women's identities were still being selected for them by a patriarchal system based on a concept of male superiority. Anger that women were still fighting for their basic human rights. The tapestry had been a vehicle I used to express what was then my deep concern for the plight of women.

Sadly, the Equal Rights Amendment was never passed, and later on, during the eighties, feminism became associated with lesbianism and a radicalism that was comparable to the labeling of witches that took place during the dark ages in Europe, and into the eighteenth century here in America. In short, feminism had been swept under the cultural rug.

My husband-to-be was pleased with this particular turn of events. In fact, Patrick, along with his cohorts in the "Christian Right," believed that feminists were evil, or, to parrot their main spokesperson, Rush Limbaugh, "feminazis."

The Christian Right, which consisted of a collective of over zealous Bible thumpers, had begun to infiltrate the political infrastructure. What this meant is that any gains women had made during the seventies and eighties were now being compromised. For example, the Christian Right did not believe women had the right to control their reproductive life; this was God's domain, in their opinion. Of course, this was the total opposite of my beliefs.

I lived with the fact that my fiancé was a staunch supporter of the Christian Right. Every month, no matter what our financial needs were, he would send money to various Christian Right groups.

Well aware of Patrick's opinions of feminism and the women's movement, I sent the "EQUAL RIGHTS AMENDMENT, 1982" tapestry to my mother immediately following the week we became engaged.

It occurred to me that the tapestry which I was now working could have very well been a proper embroidery project for a woman from the Victorian era, a woman completely devoid of opinions and of course, real passion. Depicting a simple bouquet of flowers in a vase, the tapestry utilized calm, dignified, timid colors. Certainly Patrick could find nothing objectionable about my artwork.

I turned towards Patrick, who stared intently at the television he had tuned to the Christian Broadcast Network.

"Find yourselves brothers and sisters," shouted the minister. "Turn toward Jesus Christ. Rise up, and remember..." I studied the minister's suit, which was plaid, the sort of suit you might have seen during the disco era. Perhaps it was his way of being hip within the Christian Right crowd.

"Resist the ways of Satan," the minister ranted. "Resist the Whore of Babylon. All women must obey their husbands, must *submit* or else risk letting in Satan, who will seek to destroy your entire family!"

"I can't believe this guy," I said, feeling absolutely disgusted. "He sounds like he's right out of the witch-burning days. Any minute now, he'll ask you to look for the mark of the devil. Did you know back then that anything, even a mole, was a sign of the devil?"

"*You* probably have one—don't you?" Patrick sputtered.

"You're joking, right?"

"Maybe, maybe not," Patrick retorted. "That's what baptism is for; to protect you from getting the mark of the beast."

"You're not serious," I said, but of course, I already knew the answer to my question.

"You know, right now, we could call the number at the bottom of the screen and the prayer team can pray for your lost soul," Patrick said hopefully.

"That's convenient," I said.

"Even those of you that have fallen into the devil's lair, you too can be saved. The Lord will find a way," droned the TV evangelist. "Resist the Whore of Babylon. Resist the evil power of women; do not be left behind."

I suddenly wondered if, across the nation, other women felt the same sense of shame for being born female that I did right at that moment. Then, focusing back on my tapestry, I attempted to do what is called in embroidery circles a fancy stitch, mostly because it takes a skillful use of needle and thread. At the moment, I did not appear to have any skill, because I managed to poke myself with the needle.

"Damn it," I said, nursing my nearly stitched finger. "That's the second time I've done this to myself. I guess that's why they call it crewel embroidery. It's cruel!"

Patrick, stoic, said nothing. Apparently he didn't find me amusing.

Still nursing my finger, I asked Patrick a difficult question. "How come you're so hard on women with a past?"

"Where did that come from?"

"It's just that you seem to hate women with a past, that's all," I replied meekly.

"Why do you want to know?"

I could feel my heart racing. I *had* to say something. "I, well, that is…I…"

"Spit it out."

"*I've* done some things in my past."

"No kidding," he said, grinning. "Well, I guess I figured that out."

"No, I mean, really bad things, like—"

"Look, I wasn't born yesterday. Obviously, a girl who went around penniless had to do something for money."

"I had no choice Patrick, I really didn't."

"Why don't you just tell your women friends about it. I really don't want to know any details," said Patrick, as he returned his focus back to the televised ministry still taking place.

"The Bible clearly tells us that the beast will mount the Whore of Babylon and thus the Anti-Christ will be born," proclaimed the minister. "Repent, give yourself to Christ! Join us in Heaven, before all is destroyed."

Whatever that meant, I thought. Patrick turned the TV off, and I put my tapestry down. I would be the last person to claim I'm an expert on the Bible, but I couldn't help but pick up on the misogynistic implications of what the minister had been preaching. I believed that he was trying to say that married men had better be able to control their wives, or it might bring down the end times.

Furthermore, the TV preacher was implying that if women weren't controlled, the anti-Christ would thus be born. I have always been interested in myths. In some ways, I feel I am a bit of a myth detective. Perhaps the Whore of Babylon had once been a powerful image of a Goddess that patriarchal religions relegated into a veritable she-devil. After all, ever since Eve, we women had certainly been given a bad rap.

Once again, I attempted to continue with my embroidery project, but I felt the bitter taste of feminine shame lodged deep in my throat.

* * *

"Juliet?"

"Yes."

"This is Joanne."

I sat up straight in bed. "Hey Joanne, what's up?" I said, walking into the living room so that Patrick wouldn't be able to overhear our phone call. "Are you there?" I asked, after an awkward silence.

"Juliet, oh I don't know how to say this."

"What is it? Tell me, what's wrong?"

"Denise is dead."

"What…she…she's dead?" I whispered into the phone.

"No, there must me a mistake."

"I'm afraid it's true," Joanne said somberly.

"She's really dead?"

"Her body was found a week ago."

"What the hell's going on?" Patrick called from the bedroom.

I put my hand over the receiver. "*I'll be right there.* This is a very important call." I returned my full attention to the tragic phone call. "I'm sorry, my husband…"

"I understand, it's 5 in the morning. She paused a beat. "I just had to let you know."

"Yes of course, I'm glad you called. I'm…I'm shocked. Do you have any idea what happened?"

"She was found out in the back country," Joanne said. "Out in Jamul. A little girl on horseback found her body."

"Oh my God; how horrible. *I can't believe this.* I just saw her a couple of weeks ago."

"The funeral will be on Friday morning, at the Mira Mesa Funeral Chapel."

"Does anyone know anything? Do the police know anything?"

"She had rocks in her mouth. Someone tried to bury her alive, but first they stuffed rocks in her mouth."

I suddenly felt weak, as if a five hundred pound weight had been placed square upon my shoulders. She had rocks in her mouth...I remembered that some of the women in jail had mentioned about two women, prostitutes—how they had been found with rocks in their mouths. Several of the inmates believed the police might even be involved.

Rocks in her mouth, I thought. A good girl deserves to live, a bad girl does not...

Then I remembered Denise had gone on that talk show. There were probably several people who weren't too happy about all that publicity. Such as high-profile johns who were politicians, for example, or even members of the San Diego Sheriff's department. Any number of clients might have found her need for "honesty" threatening.

"It's a terrible tragedy, Joanne...I'm afraid I'm at a loss for words."

"Yes," Joanne whispered. "It is a tragedy." I could hear the deep emotion in Joanne's voice as she fought for composure. "She will be missed."

"She changed my life," I admitted.

We said our goodbyes and promised to see each other at the funeral.

I hung up the phone. I felt both deep sadness and guilt. In the end, I had abandoned her. The very woman who had given me the opportunity to let out the secrets that had been haunting me for so long. I had *turned* from her. I had judged her. As if I was any better than her. As if I had so perfectly risen above my past and she were somehow less than...less than human. Or not human at all.

"Who the hell was that?"

"It was Joanne." Pulling myself together, I considered explaining to him that Joanne was the founder of Sex Industry

Survivors Anonymous, but quickly decided against it.

"Who's Joanne?" Patrick demanded.

"Just a friend," I said, slumping into a chair. "A friend with some very bad news."

Grumbling, Patrick came out of the bedroom. "What bad news?"

"Denise is dead. She was murdered."

He just stood there, glaring at me.

"Didn't you hear me, I said my friend is dead!"

"What happened to her?"

"Her body was found out in Jamul. In the backcountry. Her mouth was stuffed with…with—"

"With what for chrissakes," Patrick said.

"Rocks."

"Well, maybe there's a reason for that."

"What did you say?" I snapped.

"She was a *hooker*."

"So are you saying that she deserved to die?"

His silence said it all.

"Her funeral is on Friday. I'm going to go."

"Think again," Patrick said. "That's the day of our wedding rehearsal. You can't go."

"But Patrick—her funeral is in the morning and our rehearsal is not until 7 in the evening."

"I forbid you to go."

"Am I hearing you right?"

"If you go the wedding is off."

"You can't be serious."

"Oh, I couldn't be more serious," he hissed. "I've been about as open minded as I can get here, Juliet. But what would you like me to tell family members that fly in from the Mid-West? 'Oh, my bride to be is at a hooker's funeral'?"

"She was a reformed prostitute."

"Yeah, right, and I'm the pope."

"Fine," I said. "I won't go."

"Good move," Patrick said, and went back into the bedroom.

I didn't want to think. Didn't want to think about Patrick's threat. And I was numb, in a state of shock about Denise's murder. I turned on the television. Sally Jesse Raphael was hosting a panel called "Sexual Secrets: The Secret Life of American Housewives." *Honestly*, I thought. As usual, the women, who were moonlighting as escorts, made their experiences seem so glamorous.

The glamour was a lie. I turned the channel. Donahue was hosting a panel of teenaged girls who wanted to be strippers. The girls were getting a lot of attention. But the audience, despite their fascination with the girls, was also booing and hissing at them.

Prostitutes are our scapegoats. They carry our culture's unresolved sexual shame.

My friend was dead, and because of her past, if I wanted to be Patrick's wife, I could not go to her funeral. I remembered how so recently, my future husband had told me if I wanted to be a wife Denise could not be invited to our wedding.

Similarly, if I wanted to be his wife, I was forbidden to go on a talk show and discuss my past, even if I did have a wig on. Just as I had given away my tapestry, which had meant so much to me, I felt that I had to completely deny my feelings of grief over my friend's brutal death.

I had to whitewash my past, deny my sexuality, and become a blind bride waiting for permission to see.

As nervous as a Whore in Church

I am the original sin
Evil Eve
Other
Temptress
The devil's gateway
My quest?
Wholeness
To heal the sexual and the sacred.

Then,
I will be the Goddess
Isis....Artemis
Cleopatra resurrected
Cleopatra redefined
A true queen not a evil
Vamp.

The circle is broken now
Women weep
In cages
Behind veils
Prisoners
Of feminine shame.

She stands outside
Separate nonhuman
As nervous as a whore in church
Female
Responsible for the
Fall.

When I tell my story
When you tell your story
The circle will be complete
When we remember Mother, Matter and
The dignity and the grace of
The Divine Feminine Principle
The Goddess
We will be free.

chapter twenty-seven

The Second Week of December in the Last Decade of the 20th Century Downtown San Diego

I held my head high as I walked into the small funeral chapel that was located downtown, on the same street where we had held our Sex Industry Survivor's meeting. I knew Patrick had forbidden me to go to Denise's funeral, but I had to go. I would never be able to forgive myself if I didn't.

I sat in the second row from the front. I waved at Joanne, and she nodded in acknowledgement. On her right sat Denise's husband, who looked absolutely devastated. The funeral chapel's minister, in his mid-fifties and wearing a toupee, got up and began to speak.

"A lovely woman who struggled with many demons has made her transition," the minister said. "Her life has been cut short, *too* short. But out of the darkness, will always come the light," he said, as he adjusted his rug. "I know that she is in the blessed light, and that all life is immortal."

It seemed like he went on forever, and he never could get his hairpiece in the right position. Finally, the funeral proprietor stepped down, and many women of different ages and ethnic backgrounds came forward. They talked about how much Denise had meant to them, and what a difference she had made in their lives. I recognized many of the women from the jail, and one or two of the women I recognized from meetings we held at the YMCA. I also recognized a few of the guests from an accounting job Denise had worked at for a while, in between her other jobs. Some guests, who were not as buttoned-down in their appearance, were girls Denise obviously knew from the streets. But despite each woman's apparent class level, or her physical appearance, or age, we all had a common bond. Denise.

Each got up and said a few words. As I listened, I was deeply moved, and knew that I too wanted to share something about Denise. When one of the girls finished, I stood up and rushed to the podium.

"We all know Denise had difficulties with her addictions," I said, my heart pounding. "But she also had a very loving, giving, compassionate side. She did not judge you, so you became free to be who you were. She allowed me to talk about my past and thanks to her I was finally able to release the secrets I had carried inside for over a decade. Maybe this isn't the time to bring this up, but I have heard that certain members of the police force considered that her death was 'NHI' which stands for: No humans involved. When the files of victims are marked NHI, they are given low priority, if any at all."

A couple of the cops who were attending the service exchanged glances. The tension in the small chapel became as palpable as the overly fragrant smell of white gardenias.

"I don't know who killed Denise, but I do know her murder deserves just as much of an investigation as any other murder. She was *very* human, and very real," I said, my voice quavering.

"I've never met anyone like her." People were starting to cry. I paused briefly in order to regain my composure.

"Some of us do not stay here long on this planet. Some of us, I believe, are put here as teachers. Denise taught me many things. One of the most important things she taught me was that I didn't have to be ashamed of my past—that I could talk honestly about it—and that this would help me heal. Denise gave me another great gift," I said, as I placed my hand on my heart. "She helped me open up my heart, so that I could open up my throat," I said, and moved my hand from my heart to my throat.

"Whoever did this wanted to give a message—that Denise was powerless, voiceless. To get this message across the murderer placed rocks in her mouth. And yet, despite the heinous manner of these crimes, the criminal failed, because her *voice*, and her *spirit*, is eternal. Her life, and her courageous spirit to face her own dark side, will live on forever." I paused, and made eye contact with the guests at the service. Positive energy and unconditional acceptance reverberated between us. Encouraged by the warmth I felt coming towards me, I proceeded.

"The perpetrators must know that they have *not* silenced Denise. Her spirit lives on in the voices of women, who, like me, are coming forward. Denise helped form a recovery group that has already assisted women who want to get out of the sex industry.

"In time, survivors all over the world will have a place to go for help. And I think that Denise would want us to continue what she started. She would want each of us to know that we *can* help make a difference. That is the greatest gift she gave me. She helped me believe in my own ability to impact other women's lives."

And now the emotions I felt ran too deep, and so, since I had said all I needed to say, I stepped away from the podium, and I held my head high, with dignity, just as, I'm certain, Denise would have wanted me to do.

* * *

I went into the Immaculata, the church where I was soon to be married. I didn't know how I was going to grieve Denise's death. But I *had* to, or Patrick would figure out that I had been to her funeral, after all. Patrick believed that she was never supposed to be in my life in the first place. She had been a whore, so therefore she wasn't entitled to exist.

I walked down the path that led to the church. The sun was blinding—that irrepressible Southern California sunshine that sometimes could become annoying. I used the folder of papers I was carrying—my wedding vows—to shut out some of the brightness.

As well as needing a place to grieve Denise's death, I had another reason for going to the church. If I really *was* going to get married there, I wanted to try to feel comfortable. As I entered the church, I wasn't so sure that was possible. Everywhere I looked, all I could see was the struggle of Jesus Christ. Jesus on the Cross. Blood dripping through his finger tips. The wreath of thorns around his head. More blood.

I sat on a church pew. The back of the chair felt cold and hard against my back, and I knew I simply didn't belong here. Besides, how was I supposed to be comfortable with the symbols I saw here? I allowed my gaze to settle where it may, and I noticed that my attention kept returning to the beautiful statue of Mary with child.

For many years, my sister had shared her appreciation of Mother Mary with me. "But she was only a vessel," *I would argue with her.*

"That's what many religions have told us, but that's not how I see her," Marie replied.

"Go on," I said.

"I believe it was Mary who protected me all those nights when I was out there on the streets, beyond drunk sometimes," my sister Marie told me. "One night, a man, a stranger, pulled a knife on me in an alley. I proceeded

to talk to him about Mother Mary, about how she was there with me, about how much hope she gave me. All of a sudden he just dropped the knife and took off. Ever since then, I have kept images of her all around me. I have found that she gives me an incredible amount of peace."

And so as I sat here in this chilly church, reflecting back on that conversation I had shared with my sister I peered, tentatively at first, at the statue of Mother Mary. I thought of all the reports that had been made, of the sightings of Mary around the world, especially in war-torn Yugoslavia. "Pray for Peace," this Mary told the world.

I moved out of my pew and walked into a small sanctuary adjacent to the main church. There were two life-sized statues of Jesus and Mother Mary. I stood for quite some time in front of Mother Mary. I even deposited fifty cents into a small donation box in order to purchase a candle. After I lit the red candle, I watched the flame dance, and then suddenly, everything in the room became still. I looked up at Mary's face and I felt a peace, and a love that was new to me. I guess you could say I had an epiphany of some kind.

Then I grieved the loss of my friend. Denise. The whore. The bad girl. The dark side of *me*. *My shadow*. And then the tears began. In order to fit myself into the pure good/girl bride image, I had annulled my first marriage and then also attempted to whitewash my sexual past. In order to annul my first marriage, at least in the eyes of the Catholic Church, I had to admit that I was promiscuous, *an evil woman*. A drunk. I had to kill off my dark past, because I was supposed to be either a virgin or a whore. If I was unable to integrate the dark aspects of my past, then who was I? I was *still* split, *still* viewing myself through a patriarchal lens.

As I peered at the life size image of Mother Mary, I wondered if there might be another image of Mary that did not fit into a dualistic paradigm. *An image free of the either/or, Whore/Madonna dichotomy.* If only there could be another aspect of Mary that embraced the shadow aspect of ourselves, that part we tried to keep hidden. This version of the goddess would help women embrace that which we have claimed unspeakable. Abuse. Anger, and death. She would teach us to face our demons.

I pulled myself up from where I had been kneeling and I walked through the church. In the marriage I was about to enter into, I had to deny the darker aspects of my real self. Patrick did not want to hear about my past, or why it was so important for me to talk with women who had walked the path I did.

"Goodbye Denise," I said. I walked to the bowl of water that is placed by all entranceways in a Catholic church. I dipped my fingers in the water, and then made the sign of the cross.

"This blessing is for you," I whispered, "and the 45 women in San Diego who were murdered."

Then I went to one of the pews and I got down on my knees. I closed my eyes and a series of scenes played out before me. The first time I met Denise, when she openly admitted in front of a crowded AA meeting hall that she had been a prostitute. That day she took me to Los Colinas Women's Jail, and I had shared the secret I'd always thought I would take with me to the grave. That I, too, had been in the sex industry. Back then, it had been so excruciatingly painful for me to talk about my past.

It wasn't as painful for me to talk about it now. And then I remembered other meetings we had held, and the laughter, and the tears, and how I would sometimes get the chance to watch a woman open up, and let that mask crumble down. Each time they revealed themselves to me, something in me softened as well, and their honesty helped me heal and become whole.

I will never forget any of you, I thought, as I stood up. *I will never forget the women in jail, or Denise, or the 45 women who were murdered.*

Just then I noticed an elderly Hispanic woman standing in front of an image of Mother Mary. It was an image I had never seen before. This particular Mary wore a black shawl, and she was surrounded with golden light. As I walked past the elderly woman, I peered at the sign above the image she was looking at. It said, "Our Lady of Guadalupe."

Beyond her, in a small alcove on a floor above us, a beautiful chorus was practicing. Young children, their voices innocent, rang through the church.

"Hallelujah! Hallelujah," the children's voices collided with my reverie.

Just then, the woman looked away from the Madonna dressed in black and towards me. Her dark eyes were hypnotizing me; I was lost in a vortex of time and space controlled by the woman before me.

"Aloba La Diosa Negra," the elderly woman said, "Ella tiene la sabiduria."

From what I could recall from college Spanish, she had just said, *"Praise the Black Madonna,"* and that *"She has all wisdom."*

Was this, I wondered, the version of Mother Mary I had been thinking of? Was there an aspect of female divinity that I could claim as my own?

I was then struck with yet another revelation. What if all images, whether it was Jesus on the Cross, Mother Mary as Saint, or Mary Magdalene as the Prostitute, really were just keys, ways to create our own entrance to the Divine, or God?

All my life, without really knowing, I had hungered for these keys, these pathways to God. I had sought comfort in the arms of strangers, love from Greyhound bus drivers, and warmth from a father behind bars. When all along, really, I'd only been looking for God.